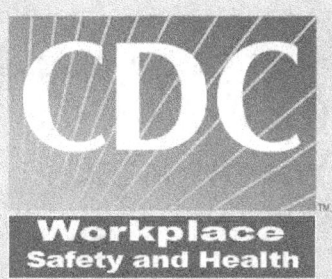

Workplace Safety and Health

Legionnaires' Disease at an Automobile and Scrap Metal Shredding Facility, New York

Randy Boylstein, MS, REHS
Rachel Bailey, DO, MPH
Chris Piacitelli, MS, CIH
Christine Schuler, PhD
Jean Cox-Ganser, PhD
Kathleen Kreiss, MD

Health Hazard Evaluation Report
HETA 2011-0109-3162
New York
August 2012

DEPARTMENT OF HEALTH AND HUMAN SERVICES
Centers for Disease Control and Prevention

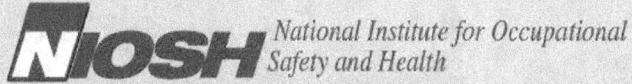 *National Institute for Occupational Safety and Health*

The employer shall post a copy of this report for a period of 30 calendar days at or near the workplace(s) of affected employees. The employer shall take steps to insure that the posted determinations are not altered, defaced, or covered by other material during such period. [37 FR 23640, November 7, 1972, as amended at 45 FR 2653, January 14, 1980].

CONTENTS

ABBREVIATIONS

CDC	Centers for Disease Control and Prevention
CFR	Code of Federal Regulations
CFU	Colony forming unit
Ct	Cycle threshold
DNA	Deoxyribonucleic acid
DFA	Direct fluorescent antibody
°F	Degrees Fahrenheit
HHE	Health hazard evaluation
mg/m³	Milligrams per cubic meter
mL	Milliliter
L.	*Legionella*
NAICS	North American Industry Classification System
NIOSH	National Institute for Occupational Safety and Health
NYSDH	New York State Department of Health
OSHA	Occupational Safety and Health Administration
PCR	Polymerase chain reaction
PEL	Permissible exposure limit
ppm	Parts per million
REL	Recommended exposure limit
VOC	Volatile organic compound

The National Institute for Occupational Safety and Health (NIOSH) received a management request in May 2011 for a health hazard evaluation at an automobile and scrap metal shredding facility in New York. Management submitted the health hazard evaluation request because four cases of Legionnaires' disease had been identified among facility workers between 2009 and 2011. Following our initial site visit, a fifth case was identified in June 2011.

What NIOSH Did

- Site visit in June 2011

  o We spoke with employees about Legionnaires' disease and any current symptoms they may have had.
  o We distributed a NIOSH-prepared handout about the health hazard evaluation and Legionnaires' disease to workers and recommended that they give the handout to their healthcare provider if they get sick.
  o We gave workers a list prepared by the local health department of healthcare providers, walk-in clinics, free clinics, and emergency departments in the area.
  o We collected air, water, and swab samples at multiple locations around the facility and tested them for *Legionella* bacteria; water samples were also tested for free chlorine content and pH.
  o We collected area air samples that were analyzed for metals, volatile organic compounds, and/or dust levels.
  o We met with health officials from the state and local health departments and reviewed medical records for known cases of Legionnaires' disease.
  o We recommended steps to decrease potential exposure to *Legionella* bacteria during our closing meeting and in a July 2011 interim letter report.

- Site visit in September 2011

  o We collected water and swab samples at multiple locations and analyzed them for *Legionella* bacteria.
  o We hung posters that showed how to put on and take off an N-95 respirator and demonstrated the procedures to some workers.
  o We posted laminated hand-washing signs in the break room and restrooms and no smoking signs in the production area.

HIGHLIGHTS OF THE NIOSH HEALTH HAZARD EVALUTION (CONTINUED)

o We recommended steps to decrease potential exposure to *Legionella* bacteria during our closing meeting.

What NIOSH Found

- Site visit in June 2011

    o Large quantities of standing water were observed throughout the facility grounds.
    o Workers stood and shoveled in or around the standing water; mobile equipment drove through puddles of water.
    o Water dripped from the exterior of the shredder and conveyors, and the shredder emitted clouds of steam.
    o Only one surface drain was visible, and water was not draining to it.
    o Shredded material on the conveyors was dirty and wet.
    o No respirators were being used.
    o *Legionella* was identified in water dripping from the exterior of the shredder onto the exit conveyor belt that contained the shredded material, and in multiple puddles of water.
    o *Legionella* was identified from a swab sample taken from a conveyor belt inside the picking shed.

- Site visit in September 2011

    o Significantly less standing water was observed on the ground.
    o A larger shredder had been installed that used less water.
    o The facility grounds had been cleared of a build-up of dirt and mud revealing a previously unseen drain, resulting in improved drainage.
    o Workers who shoveled or worked in the picking shed were wearing N-95 respirators.
    o No one wearing a respirator had been fit-tested.
    o Only the picking shed had been cleaned and sanitized.

What Managers Can Do

- Improve surface drainage to eliminate remaining standing water and continue to keep the grounds cleared of debris that inhibits drainage.

- Minimize shoveling activities in puddles of water.

- Wash and sanitize the shredder, conveyor systems, and mobile equipment twice a year.

- Perform environmental sampling for *Legionella* if another case of Legionnaires' disease is identified.

- Require mandatory use of fit-tested respirators (N-95 or higher level of protection) for workers who perform picking operations or shoveling in or around standing water, as well as for any other workers who may be exposed to aersols from pools of water, dripping or splashing water, or wet materials. Workers should also wear respiratory protection when dredging or emptying the drainage pond.

- Develop a respiratory protection program in compliance with the Occupational Safety and Health Administration respiratory protection standard, 29 Code of Federal Regulations (CFR) 1910.134.

- Workers with respiratory or flu-like symptoms should be evaluated by a healthcare provider for possible Legionnaires' disease. Signs of Legionnaires' disease can include a high fever, chills, and a cough. Some people may also suffer from muscle aches and headaches. Nausea, vomiting, and diarrhea may also occur.

What Employees Can Do

- Report respiratory or flu-like symptoms to your personal healthcare provider and, as instructed by your employer, to a designated individual at your workplace. Signs of Legionnaires' disease can include a high fever, chills, and a cough. Some people may also suffer from muscle aches and headaches. Nausea, vomiting, and diarrhea may also occur.

- Wear a fit-tested respirator when performing picking operations or shoveling in or around standing water, as well as when you may be exposed to aerosols from pools of water, dripping or splashing water, or wet materials. You should also wear respiratory protection when dredging or performing maintenance on the drainage pond.

- If your respirator gets dirty or is hard to breathe through put on a new respirator.

- Do not smoke or eat in the plant production areas.

- Always wash your hands before eating or smoking.

Five employees from the shredding facility who had performed shoveling and/or picking activities had been diagnosed with Legionnaires' disease. Upon inspection, we observed large quantities of standing water throughout the facility grounds and observed workers standing and shoveling in or around the water. *Legionella* was identified in water and swab samples collected from numerous locations around the facility. We recommended that the groundwater drainage system be improved to eliminate the pools of water, the equipment be sanitized, and workers wear N-95 respirators. Since instituting recommendations there have been no new cases.

On May 11, 2011, the National Institute for Occupational Safety and Health (NIOSH) received a request from the management of an automobile and scrap metal shredding facility regarding cases of Legionnaires' disease that had been identified among their workers. The request listed concerns about dusts, mists, and vapors generated during the process of shredding automobiles and scrap metal. The health concerns were Legionnaires' disease and respiratory disease.

During telephone discussions with the New York State Department of Health (NYSDH), NIOSH learned that four employees from the shredding facility had been diagnosed with Legionnaires' disease: one in 2009, two in 2010, and one in May 2011. All performed shoveling and/or picking activities; the latter involves manually removing copper and other material passing on a moving conveyor. In December 2010, NYSDH identified *Legionella* bacteria on a swab sample taken from a conveyor belt that exited the shredder and from water dripping from that same belt. An additional water sample obtained in May 2011 from the same conveyor belt also contained *Legionella*.

Prior to our initial site visit, NIOSH investigators contacted management and recommended that any employee with respiratory, flu-like, or gastrointestinal symptoms (e.g., fever, chills, cough, shortness of breath, muscle aches, nausea, vomiting, diarrhea) be removed from his or her job and seek evaluation for Legionnaires' disease from a healthcare provider. We also recommended that employees who work near any aerosols or mists wear fit-tested N-95 respirators.

On June 1-2, 2011, NIOSH investigators visited the facility. We spoke briefly with all available facility employees about Legionnaires' disease and any symptoms they may have or have had; none reported current symptoms consistent with Legionnaires' disease. We observed large quantities of standing water throughout the facility grounds. We also observed workers standing and shoveling in or around the water; vehicles driving through puddles of water; and front-end loaders picking up and setting down materials in and around standing water. We observed no employees wearing respirators. We collected air, water, and swab samples at multiple locations around the facility to be tested for *Legionella* bacteria. We also collected area air samples to be analyzed for metals, volatile organic compounds (VOCs) and dust. *Legionella* was identified in water dripping from the exterior of the shredder onto the exit conveyor belt that contained the shredded material and in multiple puddles of water. Metals detected in the air samples were below applicable NIOSH recommended exposure limits (RELs) and the Occupational Safety and Health Administration (OSHA) permissible exposure limits (PELs), where standards existed. Toluene, ethyl benzene and xylene isomers, and some alkyl benzenes were the major VOCs identified. The dust samples were below the OSHA particulates not otherwise regulated standard of 5 milligrams per cubic meter (mg/m³) for respirable particles.

At the end of the walk-through visit, we again recommended implementing a formal respiratory protection program that would require employees working around or near aerosols or mists to wear fit-tested N-95 respirators. We also discussed the possibility of *Legionella* in the standing water which could be aerosolized during shoveling activities and while driving or walking through the puddled water. We reiterated that symptomatic employees should be removed from their jobs until they are evaluated for Legionnaires' disease by a healthcare provider. We recommended that the groundwater drainage system be improved to eliminate the pools of water and that shoveling activities be avoided as much as possible during shredding operations because of the potential for generating aerosols. We recommended the shredder, conveyor systems, and any mobile equipment be cleaned and sanitized.

Following our initial site visit, a fifth employee was diagnosed with Legionnaires' disease in June 2011. He had recently been hired at the facility, worked in the picking shed, and had not worn a respirator.

On September 23, 2011, we revisited the facility to conduct a follow-up assessment. Facility grounds had been cleared of a build-up of dirt, improving drainage and revealing a previously blocked drain. A new shredder had been installed which required only half the previous water flow. The plant manager reported that the picking room had been cleaned and sanitized but not the rest of the facility. Some puddles of water still existed, and *Legionella* was detected in water samples taken from multiple puddles. *Legionella* was not detected in swab samples taken from the conveyor system. We observed workers wearing N-95 respirators; none had been fit-tested, and some were wearing their respirators incorrectly. In each of these cases, we showed the worker how to wear the respirator. We also hung posters in the break room and mechanical room that showed how to put on and take off an N-95 respirator. We recommended that workers wearing respirators be fit-tested. We also recommended that the ground drainage be improved to remove the remaining standing water, and that the rest of the facility be cleaned and sanitized.

Keywords: NAICS 423930 (Recycled material merchant wholesalers), Legionnaires' disease, *Legionella*, respiratory disease, personal protective equipment, PPE, water, shredding.

INTRODUCTION

On May 11, 2011, NIOSH received a health hazard evaluation (HHE) request, dated May 10, 2011, from the owner of an automobile and scrap metal shredding facility regarding cases of Legionnaires' disease that had been identified among workers. The request listed concerns about dusts, mists, and vapors generated during the process of shredding automobiles and scrap metal. The health concerns were Legionnaires' disease and respiratory disease.

BACKGROUND

In May 2011, before we received the HHE request, we had telephone discussions with the director of a regional office of the NYSDH and an industrial hygienist from the NYSDH Bureau of Occupational Health. They told us that four employees from the shredding facility had been diagnosed with Legionnaires' disease: one in 2009, two in 2010, and one in May 2011. In December 2010, upon learning of the two recent cases, the NYSDH visited the facility and collected a swab sample from a conveyor belt that exited the shredder and a sample of water dripping from that same belt; *Legionella* bacteria were identified in both samples. An additional water sample obtained in May 2011 from the same conveyor belt also contained *Legionella*. The NYSDH told us that the local county health department had been involved in investigating the cases of Legionnaires' disease since December 2010. The local county health department made several visits to the facility. They prepared a fact sheet on Legionnaires' disease which was distributed to employees and sent a letter to primary care providers in the area notifying them that employees at the shredding facility had been diagnosed with Legionnaires' disease. The letter included guidance documents from the NYSDH about Legionnaires' disease and how to diagnose it.

In April 2011, the director of the regional office of the NYSDH had sent a letter to the owner of the shredding facility and recommended that he submit an HHE request to NIOSH to assist with identifying potential environmental sources of exposure to

Legionella bacteria and recommend control methods. The director of the regional office mentioned in the letter that NIOSH might also be able to assist with evaluating fume and dust exposures at the facility. After we received the HHE request in May 2011, we contacted the shredding facility owner and his contract safety consultant. We recommended that any employee with respiratory, flu-like, or gastrointestinal symptoms (e.g., fever, chills, cough, shortness of breath, muscle aches, nausea, vomiting, diarrhea) be removed from his or her job and seek evaluation for Legionnaires' disease from a healthcare provider. We also recommended that employees working around or near any aerosols or mists wear fit-tested N-95 respirators. We discussed that this would entail instituting a formal respiratory protection program that complied with the OSHA respiratory protection standard (29 Code of Federal Regulations (CFR) 1910.134). We set dates for June 1-2, 2011 with the facility owner to visit the facility, collect environmental samples, and talk informally with employees.

We informed the staff of the local county health department and NYSDH of our initial recommendations and that we would be making the June site visit.

During the site visit in June, we also met with staff from the NYSDH and the local county health department, who provided us with medical records for the four cases. At the conclusion of the site visit at the shredding facility, we provided recommendations to the facility owner and his safety consultant.

On July 12, 2011, the NYSDH notified us that a fifth case of Legionnaires' disease had been diagnosed in a worker from the facility who had become symptomatic in mid-June 2011.

On July 13, 2011, we had a teleconference with staff from the NYSDH to review our findings and recommendations from our site visit. On July 14, 2011, we discussed the recommendations with the shredding facility's safety consultant.

On July 22, 2011, we sent an interim letter containing sample results and additional recommendations to mitigate risk of Legionnaires' disease to management of the shredding facility, their safety consultant, NYSDH, the county health department, and the OSHA regional office.

On September 23, 2011, we revisited the facility to conduct

a follow-up assessment to determine the effectiveness of any remediation work the company had undertaken following our site visit and issuing of recommendations.

Process Description

This automobile and scrap metal shredding operation covers approximately 200,000 square feet with a mix of enclosed, canopied, and open space (Figures 1a-1b). Approximately 60 workers are employed as yard men, drivers, shredder operators and laborers, eddy current workers, and office workers. Semi-trailer trucks bring scrap metal in the form of cars (pre-crushed and drained of fluids), appliances, and other items to the facility from the company's own scrap yards and a number of independent recycling operations. Trucks drive onto a scale embedded in the road for weighing, then the received material is either self-unloaded (dumped) or unloaded by mobile cranes fitted with grapples onto a large raw material pile (Figure 2). Cranes then place the material onto a conveyor belt that feeds the shredder. A large shredding machine (Figure 3) reduces the scrap metal into fist-sized pieces. An operator, stationed in a booth directly above the shredder (Figure 4), controls the flow of material through the shredder and can raise and lower the gate that controls the amount of material being fed into the shredder.

The shredder employs an electric motor to rotate a series of disks fitted with hammers inside a chamber (Figure 5). As the disk rotates, scrap is fed into the shredder where the hammers strike the material and fragment it into the smaller pieces. The shredded scrap then hits the walls of the shredder housing which contain a series of grates and passes through into the discharge unit (Figure 6). The shredding chamber is cooled and lubricated with municipal water, which is pumped into the shredding chamber by lines fitted to either side of the shredder (Figure 7). While operating, the interior of the shredding chamber can reach 500 degrees Fahrenheit (°F), so much of the water evaporates immediately in a cloud of steam, but the shredded scrap remains wet after leaving the chamber. The scrap drops onto a conveyor and is diverted into ferrous and non-ferrous process streams via magnetic separators.

In the ferrous stream, material is conveyed to a building called the "picking shed" (Figure 8), where approximately six to eight workers stand next to three conveyor lines to manually remove (pick) contaminant materials including wiring, plastic, and copper "meatballs" (pieces of copper surrounded by ferrous metal), which were included with the ferrous stream. The non-ferrous picked material is dropped into hoppers for further processing. The meatballs are diverted to a separate pile to be sold for their copper content. Depending upon ambient temperature, it was reported to us that steam is sometimes observed above the moving conveyor. After passing through the picking shed, the ferrous material is moved by conveyor belts to the ferrous pile before being loaded and shipped offsite.

The non-ferrous material, known as "fluff," is conveyed to the non-ferrous shed for further separation via eddy currents and other separation technologies and then formed into piles to await shipment offsite. Some separation of materials by manual picking also takes place on the non-ferrous side of the facility. Fluff is a complex mixture of materials including non-ferrous metal, plastics, foam, textiles, rubber, and glass.

The facility has an underground drainage system to collect waste water from the shredding and sorting processes for contaminant removal at an onsite treatment plant. Surface water flows by gravity to a nearby drainage pond (Figure 9) or enters either of two grated drains located near the shredder and near the ferrous pile and flows into an underground holding tank. The tank stores the accumulated waste water until it reaches a predetermined level which activates a pump sending the water to the waste water treatment plant. After treatment, the water is piped to a local stream.

Other buildings located on the grounds include a main office building, a maintenance garage, and an employee break room (Figures 1a-1b).

Legionnaires' Disease

Legionnaires' disease is a pneumonia (lung infection) caused by the bacterium *Legionella* which is commonly found in warm water environments and in some soils. Low natural concentrations are not generally associated with disease. The temperature range favorable for *Legionella* proliferation is 77°F–107.6°F (25°C–42°C) [ASHRAE 2000]. There are currently 54 identified species of *Legionella* [Euzeby 2012] and 70 serogroups [Fields et al. 2002]. Many *Legionella* species are known to cause health problems, with most human infections caused by *Legionella pneumophila* (L.

pneumophila) [Benin et al. 2002; Yu et al. 2009]; more than 80% of reported cases are caused by *L. pneumophila* serogroup 1 [Hilbi et al. 2010]. Other *Legionella* species [Muder and Yu 2002] known to cause human infections include: *L. micdadei* [Knirsch et al. 2000], *L. feeleii* [Sviri et al. 1997; Lee et al. 2009], *L. bozemanii* [Sobel et al. 1983; Yu et al. 2009], *L. dumoffii* [Yu et al. 2009], *L. gormanii* [Buchbinder et al. 2004], and *L. longbeachae* [Centers for Disease Control and Prevention (CDC) 2000; Whiley and Bentham 2011].

The symptoms of Legionnaires' disease are similar to other forms of pneumonia, including high fever, chills, and cough. Some may also suffer from muscle aches, headaches, nausea, vomiting, and/or diarrhea [OSHA 2011]. Symptoms usually begin two to 14 days after exposure to the bacteria. Pneumonia is confirmed either by chest x-ray or clinical diagnosis. Because the symptoms of Legionnaires' disease are nonspecific, Legionnaires' disease cannot be reliably distinguished from other forms of pneumonia on the basis of clinical presentation alone. Several laboratory tests (such as urine, sputum, and blood tests) can be used to detect the *Legionella* bacteria within the body. A commonly used diagnostic test is the urinary antigen test which evaluates a urine sample for *Legionella* antigens (foreign substances that trigger an immune system response). If the patient has pneumonia and the urinary antigen test is positive, then the patient is considered to have Legionnaires' disease [CDC 2011a]. However, the urinary antigen test only detects infections caused by *L. pneumophila* serogroup 1, but not other species or serogroups. Thus, the urinary antigen test does not permit matching with environmental samples collected during an outbreak investigation. In contrast, *Legionella* bacteria cultured from patient sputum samples can be compared to environmental isolates to more precisely document likely sources of exposure. Identification of *Legionella* infection in sputum is reduced when collection of biological samples is not performed prior to medical treatment. Blood specimens can also be used to confirm the diagnosis; a fourfold increase in antibody levels to *Legionella* bacteria in blood drawn shortly after illness and several weeks following recovery also confirm the diagnosis of Legionnaires' disease.

Outbreaks of Legionnaires' disease have been linked to a variety of warm water systems or devices that produce aerosols, sprays, or mists, such as cooling towers [García-Fulgueiras et al. 2003; Nguyen et al. 2006], whirlpool spas [Den Boer et al. 2002], decorative fountains [Palmore et al. 2009], mist machines [O'Loughlin et al. 2007], shower heads [Hanrahan et al. 1987; Darelid et al. 1994],

BACKGROUND (CONTINUED)

and industrial air scrubbers [Nygård et al. 2008]. Legionnaires' disease caused by *L. longbeachae* has been associated with soil potting mixes and composts [Steele et al. 1990; Whiley and Bentham 2011]. However, *L. pneumophila* and other species have also been found in potting soil [Casati et al. 2009; Velonakis et al. 2010] and compost [Casati et al. 2010].

Since Legionnaires' disease is a type of pneumonia it can be very serious, causing death in 5% to 30% of people identified as having the disease [CDC 2011a]. Each year, between 8,000 and 18,000 people in the United States are hospitalized with Legionnaires' disease [CDC 2011a]. Personal risk factors include age (older persons at greater risk), cigarette smoking, chronic lung disease, immunosuppression, and certain other underlying conditions (e.g., end-stage renal disease, diabetes mellitus, or cancer) [Stout and Yu 1997; CDC 2004; CDC 2011a]. The *Legionella* bacteria enter the body when bacterially contaminated mist or vapor is inhaled. Legionnaires' disease is not contagious, that is, not spread from one person to another [CDC 2011a]. Most infections can be treated successfully with antibiotics, and otherwise healthy individuals usually recover.

Legionella bacteria can also cause a milder infection called Pontiac fever. Pontiac fever is an influenza-like, self-limited illness. Symptoms may include fever, headaches, and muscle ache, last for two to five days, and usually resolve on their own [CDC 2011a]. Thus, Pontiac fever often goes undiagnosed. Pontiac fever and Legionnaires' disease may be referred to as "Legionellosis," separately or together. Legionnaires' disease and Pontiac fever are notifiable diseases. Healthcare providers and/or laboratories report cases of Legionnaires' disease and Pontiac fever to state health departments, and state epidemiologists then report those cases and other nationally notifiable diseases to the CDC.

During 2000-2009, the incidence of reported legionellosis in the United States nearly tripled from 0.39 per 100,000 persons to 1.15 per 100,000 persons [CDC 2011b]. The reasons for the increase are unknown; however, increased case detection or reporting are possible reasons for the increase [CDC 2011b]. The reported cases of legionellosis are believed to be underestimated because some cases may have been treated empirically with antibiotics and/or did not require hospitalization. Also the nonspecific symptoms of Pontiac fever likely result in substantial underdiagnoses of this form of legionellosis [CDC 2011b].

Initial site visit in June 2011

On June 1-2, 2011, NIOSH staff visited the facility. We initially met with the facility owner and his safety consultant to discuss the HHE request and our plans for the visit. NIOSH staff, the company's safety consultant, and the facility process supervisory staff then visited each aspect of operations to learn about the work flow and processes. In the early afternoon, we met with staff from the county health department to discuss the cases of Legionnaires' disease that had been identified among those who had worked at the facility and to obtain copies of medical records. The director and a public health engineer from a regional office of the NYSDH joined us at that meeting and also participated in the remainder of the walk-through later that afternoon. The facility safety consultant participated in the walk-through on both days.

We spoke briefly and individually with all available facility employees, mostly production but some office/administrative workers, about Legionnaires' disease and any current or previous symptoms they may have had. We distributed a NIOSH-prepared informational handout about the HHE at the shredding facility and Legionnaires' disease to the workers and recommended that they retain the handout to give to their healthcare provider if they get sick. Additionally, we supplied workers with the county health department's lists of healthcare providers, walk-in clinics, free clinics, and emergency departments in the area.

During the two-day walk-through visit, we collected air, water, and swab samples at multiple locations around the facility (Figure 1a) to be tested for *Legionella* bacteria. We collected air samples by pulling air at a flow rate of 12.5 liters per minute for approximately 40 to 50 minutes through an autoclaved all-glass impinger (AGI-30, Ace Glass Incorporated, Vineland, NJ) containing 20 milliliters (mL) of a 0.25% sterile yeast broth extract. The AGI-30 is a high-velocity impinger, with a stem located 30 millimeters from the bottom of the flask, that uses the principle of impingement and washing of air to trap organisms in a liquid medium [CDC 2005]. We collected samples of water in 50 mL polypropylene sterile plastic bottles. To take a swab sample, we rubbed a sterile cotton swab on a surface and then placed it in a sterile plastic bottle containing sterile distilled water. We did not measure the swabbed area or swab for a predetermined time. Onsite, we tested water samples for free chlorine content with a direct-reading digital colorimeter and for pH level with a swimming pool chlorine and pH test kit (Model 242-2, Poolmaster, Inc , Sacramento, CA). Free chlorine is the chlorine that is not currently combined with contaminants in the water. There was no rainfall on the day before or during our two-day visit.

Air, water, and swab samples were analyzed for *Legionella* by the NYSDH Wadsworth Center Laboratory. The testing involved culture of *Legionella* on agar, deoxyribonucleic acid (DNA) fingerprinting by pulsed field gel electrophoresis, and real-time *Legionella* DNA polymerase chain reaction (PCR) analyses. Samples that have the same DNA fingerprinting pattern may have a common source. In a real-time PCR assay, a positive reaction is detected by accumulation of a fluorescent signal. For each sample, cycle threshold (Ct) value 1, Ct 2, and the average Ct value were reported. Ct is defined as the number of cycles required for the fluorescent signal to cross the PCR threshold (i.e., exceed background level). Ct levels are inversely proportional to the quantity of target nucleic acid in the sample [Wisconsin Veterinary Diagnostic Laboratory 2012]; the lower the Ct value, the greater the amount of target nucleic acid in the sample. Therefore, lower Ct values indicate higher numbers of *Legionella* bacteria present while higher Ct values indicate lower numbers of *Legionella* bacteria. A difference of 3.3 Ct represents an approximate 10-fold change in concentration [Musser 2011]. A Ct value of 24 indicates approximately 200,000 bacteria/mL, while a Ct value of 33 indicates approximately 200 bacteria/mL [Musser 2011].

Since this was a new occupational setting involving *Legionella*, we attempted to gain additional perspective using a second analysis approach. Seven of the water samples were collected in duplicate. These samples were collected in 120 mL plastic bottles and sent to GTS Legionella Laboratory, a commercial laboratory in Gaithersburg, MD, to analyze using a direct fluorescent antibody (DFA) test. The DFA test uses antibodies tagged with fluorescent dye to detect the presence of *Legionella*. The laboratory concentrated the water samples 100-fold to yield a sensitivity of less than 10 colony forming unit (CFU)/mL [Gilpen 2011]. The laboratory uses a three-tiered risk approach. According to GTS, remedial action is generally not required for *Legionella* counts less than 20/mL; disinfection may be indicated (based on the location of the system and the type of employee population) for counts between 30/mL and 190/mL, and disinfection is recommended for counts between 200/mL and 1,000/mL or greater. GTS reported that when no *Legionella* is detected in a sample, this is equivalent to a culture test result of <1 CFU/mL if the culture procedure is properly performed and validated by the DFA monoclonal antibody test [GTS 2010]. GTS generally handles samples that have been collected from cooling towers, evaporative condensers, and other warm water-containing mechanical systems connected to potable or non-potable water supplies. They were unsure how samples collected from standing pools of turbid water or swabs collected from conveyor belts would fare using their methods and asked that we only send them water samples relatively free of sediment.

As there were reports of unknown fluids draining from scrap automobiles and drums brought into the facility for processing and clouds of dust and smoke generated during the shredding process, we also collected area air samples at selected locations to be analyzed for metals using NIOSH method 7303 [NIOSH 2003]. The samples were collected on 0.8 micrometer cellulose ester membrane filters at a flow rate of 2 liters per minute for approximately 200 to 300 minutes. We obtained additional area air samples for VOC screening (NIOSH method 2549) [NIOSH 2003] using thermal desorption tubes at a flow rate of 0.05 liters per minute for approximately 200 to 300 minutes; these were analyzed by thermal desorption-gas chromatography-mass spectrometry. We used a particulate monitor (pDR-1000AN personal DataRAM, Thermo Scientific Corp., Franklin, MA) to obtain real-time continuous levels of airborne dust, approximately respirable in size, as the instrument is optimized for detection of particles up to 10 micrometers. The results of the air sampling for metals and dust are time-weighted averages. We compared the results with applicable NIOSH RELs and OSHA PELs. The U.S. Department of Labor OSHA PELs (29 CFR 1910 [general industry]; 29 CFR 1926 [construction industry]; and 29 CFR 1917 [maritime industry]) are legal limits enforceable in workplaces covered under the Occupational Safety and Health Act. NIOSH RELs are recommendations based on a critical review of the scientific and technical information available on a given hazard and the adequacy of methods to identify and control the hazard. NIOSH RELs can be found in the NIOSH Pocket Guide to Chemical Hazards [NIOSH 2005].

At the end of the walk-through visit, we held a closing meeting with the owner and the facility safety consultant and discussed our preliminary findings and recommendations.

Follow-up site visit in September 2011

On September 23, 2011, we re-visited the shredding facility to conduct a follow-up assessment. The night before our visit, it had rained heavily. We collected water and swab samples at several locations that had been sampled during the first visit to be tested for *Legionella* bacteria: 1) four swab samples in sterile plastic bottles with 10 mL of sterile water added, and 2) nine water samples in duplicate. The samples were analyzed by the NYSDH Wadsworth Laboratory and GTS, as described above. For the follow-up site visit, GTS agreed to analyze swabs in addition to the water samples. For sediment-free water, GTS concentrated the water samples 100-fold to yield a sensitivity of less than 10 CFU/mL. For water samples containing sediment (e.g., dirty water), the laboratory filtered and then concentrated the water to the lowest possible volume yielding varying sensitivities (e.g., less 20, 25, 30, or 50 CFU/mL). Swab samples had the lowest sensitivity of less than 100 CFU/mL [Gilpen 2011].

We also spoke informally with workers about the use of respirators and how to properly put on and take off their respirators. We placed NIOSH informational posters about respirator usage in the workers' break room, mechanical room near the picking shed, and in the picking shed. We posted handouts in the workers' break room informing workers that since 2009, five workers at the shredding facility had been diagnosed with Legionnaires' disease. The handout also described Legionnaires' disease, how workers could protect themselves from getting Legionnaires' disease, and what to do if they felt sick. We left copies of the handout in the break room and with management. We also posted laminated hand-washing signs in the break room and restrooms and no smoking signs in the production area.

Summary of five workers with Legionnaires' disease

The five cases were all male; their mean age was 26.8 years. All were production-area workers and performed picking activities and/or shoveling in or around standing water at the time they became ill. They were employed less than one month prior to developing symptoms. Symptom onset was in April, May and June for each of three, and November for the other two. Four smoked; the other was a past smoker who lived with a smoker. Four had been hospitalized; two had been in intensive care. There were no fatalities. In addition to smoking, two had comorbidities known to be risk factors for Legionnaires' disease. All five cases were diagnosed with urinary antigen testing for *L. pneumophila* serogroup 1. Sputum was collected for culture for three of the cases; one culture was positive for *L. pneumophila* serogroup 1. In the other two cases, antibiotics had been started prior to the sputum collection, and the cultures were negative for *Legionella* growth.

Initial site visit - June 2011

Figure 1a shows the layout of the facility with sampling locations and results for *Legionella*.

In June 2011, the facility employed 63 workers: 43 in production area jobs (crane operators, loaders, maintenance, inspector, shredder groundsman, shredder operators, and laborers), 10 drivers, and 10 office and administrative staff. While at the facility, we spoke informally and individually with 41 employees and one contractor who was onsite that day, including all available production workers and some office workers. We determined that the drivers, who did not load or unload their trucks, were at little risk for exposure and did not speak with them. All production area workers were male. None of the employees with whom we spoke reported current symptoms consistent with Legionnaires' disease. More than half reported being current smokers. We talked with 15 workers who performed shoveling and/or picking activities. The laborers generally perform the picking and/or shoveling activities. Four laborers were not present on the day we talked with the workers.

Walk-through observations

We noted large quantities of standing water throughout the facility grounds (Figure 10). Workers frequently walked through the water. Debris and dirt would fall off moving conveyors. We observed workers shoveling this debris and dirt off the ground. The shoveling work often occurred in and around the standing water. We also observed workers using their shovels to scrape material out of the standing water.

Vehicles (e.g., sweeper, mobile cranes, front end loaders, Bobcats®) drove through the standing water resulting in splashing. We saw only one surface water drain in the pavement (Figure 11), between the shredder and the picking shed; it was dry while water pooled in the surrounding area. Employees reported that standing water was a problem and was not limited to after rainfall.

We observed dripping water from conveyors and occasional clouds of steam emitted from the shredder (Figure 12). The shredded material on the conveyors throughout the facility, including the picking shed, was dirty and very wet. We observed no respirator use.

The workers' break room and restroom area were orderly but very dusty and soiled. The shower stall in the restroom was used as a storage area; the shower head was missing. The break room is an allowed smoking area. Smoking is not allowed in the production areas.

Near the raw material shed, we observed a new larger shredder that was being prepared for installation in the near future (Figure 13).

Based on the walk-through observations, we again recommended implementing a formal respiratory protection program that would require employees working around or near aerosols or mists to wear fit-tested N-95 respirators. We discussed the issue of standing water in various places at the facility, the possible presence of *Legionella* in the standing water, and the potential for generation of aerosols during shoveling activities in the ferrous (near the picking shed) and non-ferrous sides of the plant and while driving or walking through puddled water. We reiterated that symptomatic employees should be evaluated by a healthcare provider for Legionnaires' disease. We provided management with copies of the informational handout that we had given to the workers. We recommended that the workers' break room and restroom be cleaned.

Environmental results

Table 1 and Figure 1a summarize the June 2011 visit results of water, swab, and air samples analyzed for *Legionella*. Six water samples (C, L, N, O, P, Q) were tested using the DFA test, *Legionella* was detected in four samples. The highest levels of *Legionella* (*L. pneumophila* and other *Legionella* species) were detected in three areas: 1) the water drainage ditch on the south side of the grounds (sample P, Figure 14); 2) in a large collection of stagnant water near the picking shed by the final ferrous pile (sample Q, Figure 15); and 3) in water dripping from the conveyor at the exit of the shredder (sample L, Figure 16).

L. pneumophila was cultured from a swab sample taken from the conveyor belt in the picking shed (sample R, Figure 17a), from water dripping from the shredder onto the conveyor belt (sample L); and in six puddles sampled. The puddles were located along the production process as follows: 1) by the raw feed pile (sample Y, Figure 18a); 2) under the shredder conveyor belt exit (sample M, Figure 16); 3) by the final ferrous pile near the picking shed (sample Q, Figure 15); 4) under a non-ferrous conveyor (sample U, Figure 19a); 5) near a non-ferrous conveyor (sample W, Figure 19a); and 6) from water drainage (towards the drainage pond) on the south side of the grounds (sample P, Figure 9). The drainage pond itself did not have culturable *Legionella*; *Legionella* bacteria were detected by the DFA test noted above. *L. pneumophila* DNA was also detected in the pond (Table 1). *L. feeleii* was cultured from water dripping from a gap between a water supply pipe and the shredder (sample A).

L. pneumophila serogroup 1 isolates that were detected in the puddle water under the shredder conveyor exit (sample M) and the puddle near the non-ferrous conveyor (sample W) had the same fingerprinting pattern (LpnS13169) and are thus considered to be related (Table 2). *L. pneumophila* serogroup 1 isolates detected in water from a puddle near the final ferrous pile (sample Q) and in water from the drainage ditch south of the shredder (sample P) had a different common pattern (LpnS13160); this same pattern was also found in a *L. pneumophila* serogroup 1 isolate detected in a sample of water dripping from the exit shredder conveyor belt collected in December 2010 by the NYSDH. This latter water sample also had a *L. pneumophila* serogroup 6 isolate with a fingerprinting pattern (LpnS13161) that matched one of two *L. pneumophila* serogroup 6 isolates detected in a swab sample taken from the exit shredder conveyor belt on the same day by the NYSDH. Samples L (*L. pneumophila* serogroups 1 and 6), R (*L. pneumophila* serogroup 6), U (*L. pneumophila* serogroup 1), and Y (*L. pneumophila* serogroup 1), and a second isolate in sample W (*L. pneumophila* serogroup 6) as well as two isolates (*L. pneumophila* serogroup 1) from a sample of water collected by the NYSDH from a conveyor belt in May 2011 had unique fingerprinting patterns (Table 2).

Using real-time PCR, *L. pneumophila*, *L. feeleii*, and other *Legionella* species were detected in multiple air, swab, and water samples taken throughout the facility (Table 1, Figure 1). Five samples (O, P, Q, U, and W), all collected from standing water, had average Ct values that ranged from 24.78 to 28.52 which correlates to roughly 200,000 to 20,000 bacteria/mL. The rest of the samples had average Ct values from 30.26 to 38.78 which would represent approximately 2,000 to virtually zero bacteria/mL.

Table 1 also includes values for pH and free chlorine concentration in water samples. The pH for all samples ranged from 7.4 to 7.8, indicating normal tap water levels. The water from the sink in the break room (sample N) and at the supply pipe for the shredder (samples A and C) had free chlorine concentrations that ranged from 0.58 to 0.77 parts per million (ppm). Water dripping from the outside of the shredder (sample L), the pond (sample O), and from puddles (samples P and Q) had free chlorine concentrations that ranged from 0 to 0.11 ppm. Most municipalities are required to keep chlorine concentration in drinking water between detectable and 4 ppm [EPA 2011].

Aluminum, barium, calcium, iron, magnesium, strontium, and zinc were detected in every air sample for metals (Table 3). Also, beryllium, cadmium, chromium, copper, lead, titanium, and vanadium were detected in some samples. All levels were well below the NIOSH RELs and OSHA PELs for those metals.

Major compounds identified from the VOC screening of area air samples were toluene, ethyl benzene and xylene isomers, and some alkyl benzenes. Other compounds identified include isopentane, trichlorofluoromethane, and various hydrocarbons. Traces of dichloro- and trichlorobiphenyl isomers and a disulfide compound were identified on some samples.

Dust measurements were collected over 200 to 300 minutes from six different locations: 1) outside grappler crane cab, 2) outside shredder operator's booth, 3) near shredder discharge, 4) inside picking shed, 5) non-ferrous shed conveyor entry area, and 6) near the drainage pond upwind of the facility (data not shown). Time-weighted average levels ranged from 0.11 mg/m^3 to 0.33 mg/m^3 at the non-ferrous shed, picking shed, and two shredder locations. A higher time-weighted average concentration of 0.83 mg/m^3 was measured at the grappler crane as it loaded materials onto the shredder conveyor. The background sample taken at the upwind location measured 0.02 mg/m^3. All samples were below the OSHA PEL of 5 mg/m^3 for respirable particulate not otherwise regulated; NIOSH does not have an applicable REL.

Follow-up after the initial site visit

On July 12, 2011, the NYSDH notified us that a fifth case of

Legionnaires' disease had been diagnosed in a worker from the facility who had become symptomatic in mid-June 2011.

On July 14, 2011, the safety consultant for the facility notified us that a respiratory protection program had been implemented at the facility around the end of June or first week of July 2011. He reported that employees working in the picking shed or shoveling under and near the picking shed were currently wearing N-95 respirators. He was unsure if the workers had been qualitatively or quantitatively fit-tested; we recommended quantitative fit-testing, as it provides a more precise indicator of the tight fit necessary to reduce the potential for leakage of outside air around the edge of the mask. We emphasized to him that all workers exposed to water, including pools of water, dripping or splashing water, or wet materials, should wear fit-tested respirators, at least until engineering control measures were implemented and evaluated for efficacy. We also discussed the environmental sample results and the need to eliminate all standing pools of water by providing proper drainage. The safety consultant told us he would share our conversation with the owner.

In August 2011, staff from the local county health department visited the shredding facility. They observed large areas of standing water. The larger shredder had been installed. The owner of the shredding facility reported that he planned to adjust the drainage at the facility. The health department staff did not observe any manual shoveling during their visit. They noted that the break room was cleaner than it had been in the past. They observed workers wearing N-95 respirators, sometimes incorrectly. They also observed workers wearing dirty and soiled N-95 respirators. The county health department recommended giving each worker a picture instruction sheet on how to properly wear and check the fitness of their respirator, as well as posting signs instructing workers to change their respirators when they become soiled and dirty or hard to breathe through. They also recommended posting signs telling workers what to do if they felt sick. The health department offered to provide the signs.

Second site visit - September 2011

The plant manager reported that the shredder and picking room had been cleaned and sanitized as recommended in our interim letter; however, the rest of the equipment had not been cleaned or sanitized. We discussed the importance of cleaning and sanitizing the entire facility and gave him a copy of our recommended cleaning and sanitizing procedure. While we were onsite, he contacted a company to schedule a time to have the entire plant cleaned and sanitized. After the site visit, the facility safety consultant notified us the cleaning and sanitizing of the facility had been completed during the last week of September.

Walk-through observations

The new larger shredder had been installed. The plant manager reported that the new shredder requires 40 gallons of water a minute for cooling and lubrication, compared to 80 gallons a minute for the old shredder. The scrap material handled by workers in the picking shed was much drier compared to the first visit (Figures 17a and b).

Dripping and standing water were much reduced (Figure 1b), even after the previous night's heavy rainstorm. The facility grounds had been cleared of a build-up of fine debris, which uncovered a blocked drain (Figure 20) near the ferrous pile and improved drainage. A smaller pool of standing water remained under the shredder conveyor; we were told that a sump pump is used regularly to pump the water from the puddle into the drainage holding tank. There was also an area of standing water between the break room and the non-ferrous shed. No plans were in place to remove or prevent the build-up of water in this area.

We observed workers who shoveled or worked in the picking shed wearing N-95 respirators. The plant manager reported that none of the workers had been fit-tested. Some workers were wearing their respirators incorrectly. In each of these cases, we showed the worker how to wear his respirator. We did not observe any hand-washing signs in the workers' break room or restrooms, non-smoking signs in the production area, or informational materials about respirators or Legionnaires' disease. We posted 1) NIOSH posters on the break room wall, mechanical room door, and in the picking shed that showed how to put on and take off an N-95 respirator (Figure 21); 2) handouts on the break room wall describing Legionnaires' disease and informing workers that since 2009 five workers had been diagnosed with Legionnaires' disease; 3) laminated hand-washing signs on the break room and restroom walls; and 4) laminated no smoking signs in the production area. We left additional copies of the handouts in the break room and with management.

We talked with the plant manager about the importance of fit-testing and informed him that this was a requirement of the OSHA Respiratory Protection Standard (29 CFR 1910.134). During our site visit, the plant manager scheduled quantitative fit-testing for the following week.

The production workers' break room and restrooms were neater and cleaner compared to our first visit.

After the site visit, the facility safety consultant notified us that fit-testing had not been completed. He reported that workers are shown how put on and take off their respirators and how to conduct a positive and negative pressure user seal check each time they wear their respirators.

Environmental results

Figure 1b shows the layout of the facility with sampling locations and results for *Legionella* from the second site visit. Table 1 presents results of water and swab samples analyzed for *Legionella*.

Legionella was not detected in any water or swab samples using the DFA test; see Table 1 for the levels of detection.

L. pneumophila was detected by culture from six of the nine water samples including: 1) water dripping from shredder onto belt (sample L, figure 16); 2) the puddle under shredder conveyor belt exit (sample M, Figure 16); 3) the puddle near shredder conveyor belt exit (sample DD, Figure 16); 4) the puddle between the break room and the non-ferrous shed (sample CC, no photo taken); 5) the drainage ditch on the south side of the grounds (sample P, Figure 14); and 6) the pond (sample O, Figure 9). *L. pneumophila* DNA was detected by PCR in water samples from all these sites, too, and in water dripping from a gap between the water supply pipe and the shredder (sample A).

L. pneumophila was not detected by culture from the four swab samples taken. The sites swabbed were: 1) the shredder exit conveyor belt (sample K); 2) a conveyor belt in the picking shed (sample R); 3) the road sweeper nozzle (sample Z); and 4) sink faucet in the break room (sample N). *L. pneumophila* DNA was detected by PCR from swab samples taken from the road sweeper nozzle and the conveyor belt in the picking shed (Table 1).

The six water samples (CC, DD, M, L, O, P) in which *L.*

pneumophila was detected by culture had average Ct values that ranged from 28.71 to 34.49 which represent approximately 20,000 (under the shredder exit conveyor belt, sample M) to almost zero bacteria/mL (in water dripping from the shredder onto the conveyor belt, sample L). There were approximately 2,000 *Legionella* bacteria/mL in the puddle near shredder exit conveyor belt (sample DD, Ct value 30.96) and in the drainage ditch south of the shredder (sample P, Ct 30.86). Sample A (water dripping from a gap between the water supply pipe and the shredder) did not grow *Legionella*; however, *Legionella* DNA was detected (Ct 35.61). The swab samples that tested positive for *Legionella* DNA (samples K, R, Z) had average Ct values that ranged from 35.29 to 36.33 (Table 1).

The samples collected during the second visit had unique fingerprinting patterns, both among themselves and compared to those from our first site visit (Table 2) and the NYSDH visits.

The pH for the water samples ranged from 6.0 to 7.0 (Table 1), in the range of normal tap water levels. The concentration of free chlorine was 0.47 ppm in water from the sink in the break room and 2.20 ppm in the road sweeper tank. The other water samples had free chlorine concentrations that ranged from 0 to 0.10 ppm.

DISCUSSION

Between January 2009 and July 2011, nine people had been diagnosed with Legionnaires' disease in the county where the shredding facility is located; the county had a population of 51,125 at the time of the 2010 census [U.S. Census Bureau 2012]. Five of those nine individuals worked at the shredding facility when they got sick, consistent with a disease cluster related to exposure at work. The purpose of this HHE was to verify that *Legionella* bacteria were present at the facility, to determine the possible sources and/or primary locations, and to suggest remediation efforts to eliminate the problem.

All of the workers who were diagnosed with Legionnaires' disease shoveled in or around the standing water and/or performed picking activities. The five cases occurred in a small subset of the workforce. Pickers and shovelers account for 30% of the current workforce. We were unable to enumerate the total number of pickers and shovelers who worked at the company in the 2009-2011 period. Despite an uncertain denominator of pickers and shovelers at risk, the occurrence of all five cases in this subgroup of employees suggests that they had a disproportionate exposure to

Legionella contaminated aerosols. At this facility, the aerosolization of puddles contaminated with *Legionella* bacteria likely resulted in exposure to *Legionella* bacteria. During our first site visit, we observed splashing of surface water when materials were dropped into it and when workers shoveled in or around standing water. Aerosolization also occurred when cranes, front-end loaders, Bobcats®, and sweepers drove though puddles of water. We also observed water dripping from wet conveyor belts and from manually and mechanically lifted wet materials.

We identified *L. pneumophila* serogroup 1 and other *Legionella* bacteria in multiple areas around the plant. Except for supply water in the break room and to the shredder and the water in the tank of the road sweeper, we identified *Legionella* bacteria by culture (which grows the *Legionella* bacteria), PCR (which detects *Legionella* DNA), or DFA (which detects *Legionella* bacteria with an antibody tagged with a fluorescent dye) in all the environmental samples collected during the our first site visit (Table 1). Some samples had higher quantities of *Legionella* bacteria than others. Based on samples that had a PCR Ct value below 28.53 or a DFA test *Legionella* count of 200/mL or greater, six samples collected during our first visit had more *Legionella* bacteria compared to the others:

1. water dripping from the shredder onto the exit conveyor belt (sample L, *L. pneumophila* serogroups 1 and 6)

2. standing water near the ferrous pile by the picking shed (sample Q, *L. pneumophila* serogroup 1)

3. standing water near a non-ferrous conveyor (sample W, *L. pneumophila* serogroups 1 and 6)

4. standing water under a non-ferrous conveyor (sample U, *L. pneumophila* serogroup 1)

5. drainage area with standing water south of the shredder (sample P, *L. pneumophila* serogroup 1)

6. drainage pond (sample O, no culture growth)

A limitation of PCR and the DFA test is that they cannot differentiate between living and dead organisms and may give false negative results [Hung et al. 2005]. Of the six samples noted above, the first five samples (L, Q, W, U, and P) had positive *Legionella* cultures, showing the presence of living bacteria. Four additional samples during our first visit also had positive *Legionella* cultures:

1. standing water by the raw feed pile
   (sample Y, *L. pneumophila* serogroup 1)

2. water dripping from gap between
   water supply pipe and shredder
   (sample A, *L. feeleii*)

3. standing water under the shredder conveyor belt exit
   (sample M, *L. pneumophila* serogroup 1)

4. conveyor belt in the picking shed
   (sample R, *L. pneumophila* serogroup 6)

The laboratory results showed the absence or presence of *Legionella* growth, the *Legionella* species, as well as serogroup 1 or 6 for *L. pneumophila*. However, the test results did not show the concentration or quantity of bacteria that was cultured, so we were unable to evaluate the potential amplification of *Legionella* in the samples. Samples M and W had the same DNA fingerprinting pattern for *L. pneumophila* serogroup 1, suggesting a common source; similarly, samples P and Q and a sample collected previously by the NYSDH had different identical fingerprinting patterns. All other samples had unique patterns, suggesting multiple sources of *Legionella*.

During our first visit in June 2011, the drainage system was inadequate, as could be seen by the numerous pools of standing water and wet dirt on the asphalt and concrete areas throughout the facility. During our second visit, there was significantly less water on the ground, and most of the dirt had been removed (Figures 22 to 24). Also a larger shredder had been installed that used less water, resulting in less water dripping onto the ground during the shredding process. However, some standing water still existed. *Legionella* was cultured from four puddles (samples CC, DD, M, and P), the drainage pond (sample O), as well as from water dripping from the shredder onto the conveyor belt (sample L). As before, we could not determine the concentration or quantity of *Legionella* bacteria that was cultured; however, the PCR average Ct values in the water samples with *Legionella* growth for the second visit ranged from 28.71 to 34.49 indicating approximately 20,000 *Legionella* bacteria/mL (in the puddle under the shredder exit conveyor belt) to almost zero *Legionella* bacteria/mL (in water dripping from the shredder onto the conveyor belt). The DFA test was below the limit of detection for all the samples; however, the sensitivity varied among the samples. For sediment-free water, GTS concentrated the water samples 100-fold to yield a sensitivity of less than 10 CFU/mL. For water samples containing sediment (e.g., dirty water), the laboratory filtered, then concentrated the water to the lowest possible volume yielding varying sensitivities (e.g., less 20, 25, 30, or 50 CFU/mL). Swab samples had the lowest sensitivity of less than 100 CFU/mL [Gilpen 2011]. The fingerprinting patterns were different than the patterns identified during our first visit and from the NYSDH samples, indicating various sources of *Legionella* bacteria.

We do not believe the shredder was a source of *Legionella*. In the shredder itself, low concentrations of *Legionella* DNA were detected in samples taken during our first visits; however, *Legionella* was not cultured from these samples. The high temperatures inside the shredder during operation are not conducive to the growth of the bacteria. The interior of the shredding chamber can reach 500°F, and most of the water evaporates during the shredding operation and produces a plume of steam above and around the shredder.

Although a large portion of the standing water has been removed, the rest of the standing water needs to be removed to reduce the potential for exposure to *Legionella*. Standing water when heated by sunlight is an ideal environment for *Legionella* growth [OSHA 1999]. *L. pneumophila* has been isolated in puddles of rainwater on asphalt roads, especially during warm weather [Sakamoto et al. 2009]. When standing water at the shredding facility is disturbed, workers are at risk for exposure to *Legionella* bacteria. The free chlorine content of the water from puddles was low relative to the water entering the shredder. Free chlorine is the chlorine that is not currently combined with contaminants in the water. In other words, it is not occupied and still available (measurable) in the water. The relatively low free chlorine measured in the puddles could be attributed to the proportion of the puddles from rainwater (and thus absent of chlorine) and/or water from the shredding operation which may have lost available free chlorine due to interaction with oil, dirt, debris, and heat.

Because standing water still exists and there is potential for aerosolization of water contaminated with *Legionella* bacteria, we recommend that workers who perform picking operations or shoveling in or around standing water, as well as any other workers exposed to pools of water, dripping or splashing water, or wet materials wear fit-tested N-95 respirators. In addition to removing the standing water and wearing respirators, we also recommend that the equipment at the facility be cleaned and sanitized twice a year. This is necessary to remove any biofilm (containing

DISCUSSION (CONTINUED)

Legionella bacteria) on the equipment. In cooling towers, traditional oxidizing agents such as chlorine and bromine have proven effective in controlling *Legionella* [OSHA 1999; ASHRAE 2000]. At this facility, we recommended in our interim letter a mixture of regular unscented household bleach (5.25% chlorine as sodium hypochlorite) with water at a concentration of 65 to 200 ppm (see recommendations below) for the sanitization process. Because chlorine loses its effectiveness quickly in the presence of oil, dirt, and organic material [OSHA 1999], we recommended a cleaning step with a detergent solution to remove excess dirt before the sanitizing treatment (with the bleach solution). Scrubbing is necessary during the cleaning step to remove any biofilm containing *Legionella* bacteria. Periodic cleaning and sanitizing of the equipment will likely be necessary to reduce the nutrients available for *Legionella* regrowth. Because aerosols may be generated during the cleaning and sanitizing process, respiratory protection for workers engaged in cleaning is critical to preventing legionellosis.

All dust concentrations were below the OSHA PEL of 5 mg/m^3 for respirable particulate not otherwise regulated. Although NIOSH does not have a REL for respirable particulate matter to compare with, all samples for metals in the dust were found to be below both NIOSH and OSHA guidelines. The samples collected on the first site visit for a VOC screening detected toluene (a common solvent), ethyl benzene (a paint ingredient), trichlorofluoromethane (refrigerant), and a variety of other solvents and chemical components of materials used in the manufacturing of automobiles and appliances. Detection of these VOCs by the highly sensitive analytical method indicates presence of the compounds but cannot indicate levels of actual exposure.

CONCLUSIONS

Legionnaires' disease is generally considered to be preventable because controlling or eliminating the bacterium in certain reservoirs will prevent cases of the disease. No new cases of Legionnaires' disease have been identified in workers from this facility since standing water was reduced, equipment was cleaned and sanitized, and respiratory protection was implemented.

In this type of industrial setting, standing water can be aerosolized, resulting in potential exposure to *Legionella* bacteria. Legionnaires' disease should be considered when persons who work in industrial settings around standing water with potential for aerosolization present with an acute febrile respiratory illness with systemic symptoms.

RECOMMENDATIONS

Based on our findings, we recommend the following actions to create a more healthful workplace. We encourage you to use these recommendations to develop an action plan based, if possible, on the "hierarchy of control" approach. This approach groups actions by their likely effectiveness in reducing or removing hazards. In most cases, the preferred approach is to first eliminate hazardous materials or processes and, secondly, to install engineering controls to reduce exposure or shield employees. Until such controls are in place, or if they are not effective or feasible, administrative measures and/or personal protective equipment may be needed.

Eliminating hazards

1. Continue to maintain the outdoor ground surface area of the facility so the surface water drainage system can eliminate all stagnant/standing pools of water.

2. Fill in the depression under the shredder (Figure 16) so water will flow to the drainage grate rather than using a sump pump to remove the water. This would be a more permanent solution and would prevent the accumulation of water in this area. Until then, ensure that the sump pump is used under a rigidly enforced daily schedule.

3. Improve drainage to prevent pooling of water in the area between the non-ferrous building and the break room to improve drainage.

4. Continue to maintain the integrity of the drainage system to assist in the elimination of run-off water.

Engineering controls and work practices

5. Minimize shoveling activities in puddles of water as much as possible.

6. Twice a year, wash and sanitize the shredder, conveyor systems, and mobile equipment.

    a). Scrub the equipment with brushes and a detergent solution.

    b). Rinse off the equipment with water to remove the detergent and any oil, dirt, and debris. Avoid the used of high-pressure power washers or other cleaning equipment that create aerosols.

c). Mix regular unscented household bleach (5.25% chlorine as sodium hypochlorite) with water at a concentration of 65 to 200 ppm.

Amount of 5.25% sodium hypochlorite bleach	Amount of water	Concentration of bleach solution
One teaspoon	One gallon	65 ppm
One tablespoon	One gallon	200 ppm

d). Put the bleach and water solution into a container and spray the solution onto the equipment surfaces and allow the solution to sit on the equipment for approximately 10-20 minutes. Prior to this step, check with the manufacturers of your equipment to determine if a bleach solution* would damage the equipment.

*The recommended pH level for an effective and safe sanitizing solution is 6.5 to 7.5. Solutions with pH greater than 8 lose their sanitizing effectiveness, while solutions with a pH lower than 6 are more corrosive and may potentially damage equipment. Potentially harmful levels of chlorine gas may be generated if the pH of the solution is lower than 5 [McGlynn 2004]. Never mix bleach or bleach-containing products with ammonia or ammonia-containing products.

e). Scrub the equipment surfaces with brushes.

f). Rinse off the equipment with water to remove the bleach solution.

7. Avoid the release of highly chlorinated water into the drainage pond and stream as this could be a violation of environmental standards because of its detrimental effects to living organisms.

8. Personnel cleaning and sanitizing the equipment should be trained in the cleaning/sanitizing procedure and wear personal protective equipment:
   a). Eye protection (goggles or a full-face respirator)
   b). Gloves (natural rubber, neoprene, nitrile, polyvinyl chloride, or polyurethane)
   c). Respirator with a high-efficiency particulate air filter and chemical cartridge

9. Perform environmental sampling for *Legionella* if another case of legionellosis is identified.

10. Regularly clean the workers' break room and restroom.

Respiratory Protection

11. Require mandatory use of respirators (at least at the N-95 level of protection) for workers who perform picking operations or shoveling in or around standing water, as well as for any other workers who may be exposed to pools of water, dripping or splashing water, or wet materials. Workers should also wear respiratory protection when dredging or emptying the drainage pond.

12. Ensure workers wear fit-tested respirators (after they have been medically cleared). Appendix A of the OSHA respiratory protection standard details the mandatory fit-test protocols (found in appendix A of this report). Qualitative fit-testing may be used for negative-pressure air-purifying respirators, which must achieve a fit factor of 100 or less (such as the N-95 respirators which have a fit factor of 10). In contrast, quantitative fit-testing is an appropriate approach for all classes of respirators. For tight-fitting respirators (such as an N-95 respirator) also ensure that workers perform a "user seal check" (positive and negative pressure checks) each time they wear their respirator. The procedure is outlined in appendix B1 of the OSHA respiratory protection standard (found in appendix B of this report).

13. Workers should change their N-95 respirator when it becomes dirty or hard to breathe through.

14. Develop a respiratory protection program. The OSHA respiratory protection program includes the following elements:

    a). Written policy.
    b). Change-out schedule for cartridges/filters.
    c). Medical evaluation prior to use to determine fitness.
    d). Fit-testing and training prior to use and annually.
    e). Establishment and implementation of procedures for proper respirator use, such as: prohibiting use with facial hair when this would impair the seal; ensuring user seal-check and inspection of respirators prior to each use; ensuring proper cleaning, disinfection, and maintenance of respirators; and ensuring proper storage of respirators to protect respirators from damage, contamination, dust, sunlight, and extreme temperatures.

RECOMMENDATIONS
(CONTINUED)

Details about the OSHA Respiratory Protection Standard (29 CFR 1910.134) are available at http://www.osha.gov/pls/oshaweb/owadisp.show_document?p_table=STANDARDS&p_id=12716

Information about respirators can be found on the NIOSH website at http://www.cdc.gov/niosh/topics/respirators/

Hazard Communication

15. Ensure that workers understand the hazards associated with working at the shredding facility and how to protect themselves. OSHA's Hazard Communication Standard (29 CFR 1910.1200), also known as the "Right to Know Law," requires that employees are informed and trained about potential work hazards and associated safe practices, procedures, and protective measures. In your facility, workers should understand the symptoms and potential seriousness of Legionnaires' disease and the importance of seeking appropriate medical attention when ill, including informing their healthcare provider of the legionellosis risk.

Medical surveillance

16. Workers should report respiratory or flu-like symptoms to their personal healthcare provider and, as instructed by their employer, to a designated individual at your workplace.

17. Workers with respiratory or flu-like symptoms should be evaluated by a healthcare providers for possible Legionnaires' disease. Signs of Legionnaires' disease can include a high fever, chills, and a cough. Some people may also suffer from muscle aches and headaches. Nausea, vomiting, and diarrhea may also occur.

18. Do not smoke or eat in the plant production areas. Always wash hands before eating or smoking. Smoking causes many diseases and reduces the health of smokers in general, and smoking itself increases the chances that a person will develop Legionnaires' disease if that person is exposed to *Legionella* bacteria. We recommend implementing a smoking cessation program to assist employees to stop smoking.

REFERENCES

American Society of Heating, Refrigeration and Air-conditioning Engineers (ASHRAE) [2000]. ASHRAE guideline 12-2000, Minimizing the risk of legionellosis associated with building water systems.

Benin AL, Benson RF, Besser RE [2002]. Trends in legionnaires' disease, 1980-1998: declining mortality and new patterns of diagnosis. Clin Infect Dis. 35(9):1039-46.

Buchbinder S, Leitritz L, Trebesius K, Banas B, Heesemann J [2004]. Mixed lung infection by *Legionella pneumophila* and *Legionella gormanii* detected by fluorescent in situ hybridization. Infection. 32:242-5.

Casati S, Gioria-Martinoni A, Gaia V [2009]. Commercial potting soils as an alternative infection source of *Legionella pneumophila* and *Legionella* species in Switzerland. Clin Microbiol Infect. 15:571–5.

Casati S, Conza L, Bruin J, Gaia V [2010]. Compost facilities as a reservoir of *Legionella pneumophila* and other *Legionella* species. Clin Microbiol Infect. 16:945-7.

Centers for Disease Control and Prevention (CDC) [2000]. Legionnaires' disease associated with potting soil–California, Oregon, and Washington, May-June 2000. MMWR Morb Mortal Wkly Rep. Sep 1;49(34):777-8.

CDC [2004]. Guidelines for preventing health-care-associated pneumonia, 2003: recommendations of CDC and the healthcare infection control practices advisory committee. **MMWR Morb Mortal Wkly Rep.** 53(No. RR-3).

CDC [2005]. Procedures for the recovery of *Legionella* from the environment. Atlanta GA: U.S. Department of Health and Human Services, Centers for Disease Control and Prevention. http://www.cdc.gov/legionella/files/legionellaprocedures-508.pdf.

CDC [2011a]. Patient facts: learn more about Legionnaires' disease. Legionellosis Resource Site (Legionnaires' Disease and Pontiac Fever). http://www.cdc.gov/legionella/patient_facts.htm. Date accessed: August 2012.

CDC [2011b]. Legionellosis — United States, 2000-2009. MMWR Morb Mortal Wkly Rep. Aug 19;60(32):1083-6.

CFR. Code of Federal Regulations. Washington, DC: U.S. Government Printing Office, Office of the Federal Register.

Darelid J, Bengtsson L, Gästrin B, Hallander H, Löfgren S, Malmvall BE, Olinder-Nielsen AM, Thelin AC [1994]. An outbreak of Legionnaires' disease in a Swedish hospital. Scand J Infect Dis. 26:417-25.

References (CONTINUED)

Den Boer JW, Yzerman EP, Schellekens J, Lettinga KD, Boshuizen HC, Van Steenbergen JE, Bosman A, Van den Hof S, Van Vliet HA, Peeters MF, Van Ketel RJ, Speelman P, Kool JL, Conyn-Van Spaendonck MA [2002]. A large outbreak of Legionnaires' disease at a flower show, the Netherlands, 1999. Emerg Infect Dis. 8:37-43.

Environmental Protection Agency (EPA) [2011]. Basic information about disinfectants in drinking water: chloramine, chlorine and chlorine dioxide. http://water.epa.gov/drink/contaminants/basicinformation/disinfectants.cfm. Date accessed: August 2012.

Euzeby JP. List of prokaryotic names with standing in nomenclature—genus Legionella. http://www.bacterio.cict.fr/l/legionella.html. Date accessed: August 2012.

Fields BS, Benson RF, Besser RE [2002]. Legionella and Legionnaires' disease: 25 years of investigation. Clin Microbiol Rev. 15:506–26.

García-Fulgueiras A, Navarro C, Fenoll D, García J, González-Diego P, Jiménez-Buñuales T, Rodriguez M, Lopez R, Pacheco F, Ruiz J, Segovia M, Balandrón B, Pelaz C [2003]. Legionnaires' disease outbreak in Murcia, Spain. Emerg Infect Dis. 9:915–21.

Gilpen, R. (gilpen@legionella.com) [2011]. Sampling sensitivity. E-mail message to Randy Boylstein (zig1@cdc.gov), October 3.

GTS Legionella Laboratory [2010]. Laboratory Test Request and Information. http://www.legionella.com/index.html. Date accessed: August 2012.

Hanrahan JP, Morse DL, Scharf VB, Debbie JG, Schmid GP, McKinney RM, Shayegani M [1987]. A community hospital outbreak of legionellosis. Transmission by potable hot water. Am J Epidemiol. 125:639-49.

Hilbi H, Jarraud S, Hartland E, Buchrieser C [2010]. Update on Legionnaires' disease: pathogenesis, epidemiology, detection and control. Mol Microbiol. 76:1-11.

Hung LL, Miller JD, Dillon HK, eds. [2005]. Field guide for the determination of biological contaminants in environmental samples. 2nd ed. Fairfax, VA: American Industrial Hygiene Association, pp. 129–40.

Knirsch CA, Jakob K, Schoonmaker D, Kiehlbauch JA, Wong SJ, Della-Latta P, Whittier S, Layton M, Scully B [2000]. An outbreak of Legionella micdadei pneumonia in transplant patients: evaluation, molecular epidemiology, and control. Am J Med. 108:290–295.

Lee J, Caplivski D, Wu M, Huprikar S [2009]. Pneumonia due to Legionella feeleii: case report and review of the literature. Transpl Infect Dis. 11:337–40.

References (continued)

McGlynn W [2004]. Guidelines for the use of chlorine bleach as a sanitizer in food processing operations. Oklahoma Cooperative Extension Service, Division of Agricultural Science and Natural Resources. http://pods.dasnr.okstate.edu/docushare/dsweb/Get/Document-963/FAPC-116web.pdf. Date accessed: August 2012.

Muder RR, Yu VL [2002]. Infection due to *Legionella* species other an *L. pneumophila*. Clin Infect Dis. 35:990-8.

Musser K (musser@wadsworth.org) [2011]. PCR Ct values. E-mail message to Randy Boylstein (zig1@cdc.gov), July 14.

National Institute for Occupational Safety and Health (NIOSH) [2003]. In: Schlecht P, O'Connor P, eds. Manual of Analytical Methods (NMAM), 4th ed., Third Supplement. Cincinnati, OH: U.S. Department of Health and Human Services, DHHS (NIOSH) Publication No. 2003-154. http://www.cdc.gov/niosh/docs/2003-154/method-i.html.

NIOSH [2005]. NIOSH pocket guide to chemical hazards. Cincinnati, OH: U.S. Department of Health and Human Services, Centers for Disease Control and Prevention, National Institute for Occupational Safety and Health, DHHS (NIOSH) Publication No. 2005-149. http://www.cdc.gov/niosh/npg/. Date accessed: August 2012.

Nygård K, Werner-Johansen O, Ronsen S, Caugant DA, Simonsen O, Kanestrom A, Ask E, Ringstad J, Ødegård R, Jensen T, Krogh T, Høiby EA, Ragnhildstveit E, Aaberge IS, Aavitsland P [2008]. An outbreak of Legionnaires' disease caused by long-distance spread from an industrial air scrubber in Sarpsborg, Norway. Clin Infect Dis. 46:61–9.

Nguyen TM, Ilef D, Jarraud S, Rouil L, Campese C, Che D, Haeghebaert S, Ganiayre F, Marcel F, Etienne J, Desenclos JC [2006]. A community-wide outbreak of Legionnaires disease linked to industrial cooling towers--how far can contaminated aerosols spread? J Infect Dis. 193:102-11.

O'Loughlin RE, Kightlinger L, Werpy MC, Brown E, Stevens V, Hepper C, Keane T, Benson RF, Fields BS, Moore MR [2007]. Restaurant outbreak of Legionnaires' disease associated with a decorative fountain: an environmental and case–control study. BMC Infect Dis. 7:93.

Occupational Safety and Health Administration (OSHA) [1999]. Legionnaires' disease. In: OSHA technical manual. Washington, DC: U.S. Department of Labor, Occupational Safety and Health Administration, DOL (OSHA) Directive TED 01-00-015 [TED 1-0.15A]. http://www.osha.gov/dts/osta/otm/otm_iii/otm_iii_7.html. Date accessed: August 2012.

Occupational Safety and Health Administration (OSHA) [2011]. Section I: what is Legionnaires' disease? eTools Home: Legionnaires' Disease. http://www.osha.gov/dts/osta/otm/legionnaires/disease_rec.html#Causative. Date accessed: August 2012.

REFERENCES (CONTINUED)

Palmore TN, Stock F, White M, Bordner M, Michelin A, Bennett JE, Murray PR, Henderson DK [2009]. A cluster of cases of nosocomial Legionnaires' disease linked to a contaminated hospital decorative water fountain. Infect Control Hosp Epidemiol. 30:764-8.

Sakamoto R, Ohno A, Nakahara T, Satomura K, Iwanaga S, Kouyama Y, Kura F, Kato N, Matsubayashi K, Okumiya K, Yamaguchi K [2009]. *Legionella pneumophila* in rainwater on roads. Emerg Infect Dis. 15:1295-7.

Sobel JD, Krieger R, Gilpin R, Griska L, Agarwal P [1983]. *Legionella bozemanii*. Still another cause of pneumonia. 250:383-5.

Steele TW, Lanser J, Sangster N [1990]. Isolation of *Legionella longbeachae* serogroup 1 from potting mixes. Appl Environ Microbiol. 56:49–53.

Stout JE, Yu VL [1997]. Legionellosis. N Engl J Med. 337:682–7.

Sviri S, Raveh D, Boldur I, Safadi R, Libson E, Ben-Yehuda A [1997]. *Legionella feeleii* pneumonia and pericarditis. J Infect. 34:277-9.

U.S. Census Bureau [2012]. State and county quickfacts. http://quickfacts.census.gov/qfd/states/. Date accessed: August 2012.

Velonakis EN, Kiousi IM, Koutis C, Papadogiannakis E, Babatsikou F, Vatopoulos A [2010]. First isolation of *Legionella* species, including *L. pneumophila* serogroup 1, in Greek potting soils: possible importance for public health. Clin Microbiol Infect. 16:763-6.

Wisconsin Veterinary Diagnostic Laboratory [2012]. Real Time PCR Ct Values. http://www.wvdl.wisc.edu/PDF/WVDL.Info.PCR_Ct_Values.pdf. Date accessed: August 2012.

Whiley H, Bentham R [2011]. *Legionella longbeachae* and legionellosis. Emerg Infect Dis. 17:579-83.

Yu H, Higa F, Koide M, Haranaga S, Yara S, Tateyama M, Li H, Fujita J [2009]. Lung abscess caused by *Legionella* species: implication of the immune status of hosts. Intern Med. 48:1997-2002.

TABLES

Table 1. Results of air, water, and swab samples collected for *Legionella* analyses by culture, real-time polymerase chain reaction (PCR) and direct fluorescent antibody (DFA) test at a shredding facility, New York, June and September 2011

Sample type	Sample ID*	Location	Sub-location	Culture† L. pneumophila with Serogroup identification	PCR‡ L. species DNA	PCR‡ L. pneum. DNA	PCR‡ L. feeleii DNA	DFA§ L. species	DFA§ L. pneum	Water sample pH	Water sample Free chlorine (ppm)¶
First site visit (June 1-2, 2011)											
Air	A-01	Shredder	Upper level	–	–	+	–	·	·	·	·
	A-02	Shredder	Pin puller	–	–	+	–	·	·	·	·
	A-03	Non-ferrous	Central	–	–	+	–	·	·	·	·
	A-04	Non-ferrous-Under corner	Near conveyor	–	–	+	–	·	·	·	·
	A-05	Picking shed (outside)	Under stairs, near monitor screen	–	–	+	–	·	·	·	·
	A-06	Picking shed (inside)	On wall, middle area, next to door	–	–	+	–	·	·	·	·
	A-07	Blank	Blank	–	–	–	–	·	·	·	·
Swab	B	Shredder-Inside	Water nozzle, north side	–	–	+	–	·	·	·	·
	C	Shredder-Inside	Water nozzle, south side	–	–	+	–	·	·	·	·
	D	Shredder-Inside	Upper portion, east side	–	–	+	–	·	·	·	·
	E	Shredder-Inside	Lower ledge, east side	–	–	+	–	·	·	·	·
	F	Shredder-Inside	Above feed roll, west side	–	+	–	–	·	·	·	·
	G	Shredder-Inside	Feed roll, west side	–	+	–	–	·	·	·	·
	H	Shredder-Inside	Chute, west side	–	+	–	–	·	·	·	·
	I	Shredder-Inside	Base of lift piston, south side	–	–	+	–	·	·	·	·
	J	Shredder-Exit conveyor	North side	–	–	+	–	·	·	·	·
	K	Shredder-Exit conveyor	South side	–	+	–	–	·	·	·	·
	N	Break room	Sink faucet	–	–	–	–	·	·	·	·
	R	Picking shed-Conveyor	Conveyor belt	6	inc @	inc @	–	·	·	·	·
	S	Drain	Fluff pile	–	–	+	–	·	·	·	·
	T	Non-ferrous-Conveyor	Conveyor belt	–	–	+	–	·	·	·	·
	V	Non-ferrous Conveyor	Conveyor belt	–	+	–	–	·	·	·	·
	X	Eddy current-Conveyor	Conveyor belt	–	+	–	–	·	·	·	·
	Z	Road sweeper	Nozzle	–	–	+	–	·	·	·	·
	Blank	Distilled water	Distilled water for swabs	–	–	–	–	·	·	·	·
Water	A	Shredder-Outside	Water dripping from gap between water supply pipe and shredder	*Feeleii* **	+	–	+	·	·	7.6	0.65
	C	Shredder-Inside	Water nozzle, south side	–	–	–	–	<10	<10	7.6	0.58

Tables (continued)

Table 1. (cont.) Results of air, water, and swab samples collected for *Legionella* analyses by culture, real-time polymerase chain reaction (PCR) and direct fluorescent antibody (DFA) test at a shredding facility, New York, June and September 2011

Sample type	Sample ID*	Location	Sub-location	Culture† L. pneumophila with Serogroup identification	PCR‡ L. species DNA	PCR‡ L. pneum. DNA	PCR‡ L. feeleii DNA	DFA§ L. species	DFA§ L. pneum	Water sample pH	Water sample Free chlorine (ppm)¶
	L	Shredder-Exit conveyor	Dripping from shredder onto belt	1,6	–	+	–	400	200	7.6	0
	M	Puddle	Under shredder conveyor belt exit	1	–	+	–	.	.	.	.
	N	Break room	Sink faucet	–	–	–	–	10	<10	.	0.77
	O	Pond	Pond	–	–	++	–	60	80	7.4	0.01
	P	Puddle	Drainage ditch south of shredder	1	–	++	–	600	800	7.8	0.04
	Q	Puddle	Ferrous pile	1	–	++	–	400	600	7.8	0.11
	U	Puddle	Under non-ferrous conveyor	1	–	++	–	.	.	.	.
	W	Puddle	Near non-ferrous conveyor	1,6	–	++	–	.	.	.	.
	Y	Puddle	Raw feed pile	1	–	+	–	.	.	.	.
Second site visit (September 23, 2011)											
Water	BB	Road sweeper	Tank	–	–	–	–	<10	<10	7.0	2.20
	N	Break room	Sink faucet	–	–	–	–	<10	<10	6.5	0.47
	CC	Puddle	Between non-ferrous shed and breakroom	3	–	+	–	<30	<30	7.0	0.10
	DD	Puddle	Near shredder conveyor belt exit	1	–	+	–	<50	<50	6.5	0
	M	Puddle	Under shredder conveyor belt exit	1	–	++	–	<100	<100	6.5	0.07
	A	Shredder-Outside	Water dripping from gap between water supply pipe and shredder	–	–	+	–	<10	<10	6.0	0.01
	L	Shredder-Exit conveyor	Dripping from shredder onto belt	3	–	+	–	<20	<20	7.0	0.02
	P	Puddle	Drainage ditch south of shredder	1,6	–	+	–	<100	<100	7.0	0.06
	O	Pond	Pond	1,3,6,12,††	–	+	–	<25	<25	6.5	0.10
Swab	Z	Road sweeper	Nozzle	–	–	+	–	<100	<100	.	.
	N	Break room	Sink faucet	–	–	–	–	<100	<100	.	.
	K	Shredder-Exit conveyor	South side	–	+	–	–	<100	<100	.	.
	R	Picking shed-Conveyor	Conveyor belt	–	–	+	–	<100	<100	.	.

*Bold sample IDs indicate samples that were taken at similar locations during both visits.

†A number in this column indicates a positive finding of that serogroup type, a negative (-) sign indicates a negative test.

‡If *L. pneumophila* DNA was solely detected then a positive sign is only notated in that column and not in L. species column. Ct value: number of cycles before sample crosses PCR threshold. In general, lower Ct values indicate higher numbers of *Legionella* bacteria while higher Ct values indicate lower numbers of *Legionella* bacteria/mL. Specifically, a Ct of 24 is approximately 200,000 bacteria/mL while a Ct of 33 is approximately 200 bacteria/mL, with every difference of 3.3 Ct being a 10-fold change in the concentration [Musser 2011]. A negative sign (–) means DNA was not detected; one plus sign (+) indicates average Ct value was between 30.25 and 38.79; two plus signs (++) indicates average Ct value was between 24.77 and 28.72.

§ A dot (.) indicates no sample was taken, a < sign indicates result below the limit of detection, and a number represents *Legionella* CFU/mL.

¶ A dot (.) indicates no sample was taken.

** Only *L. feelei* was found in this sample; @ indicates inconclusive result.

†† Sero undetermined.

Table 2. DNA fingerprinting patterns of cultured *Legionella* bacteria

Sample ID	Location	Sub-location	Organism Cultured*	Fingerprinting Pattern
New York State Department of Health visit (December 16, 2010)				
1	Shredder-Conveyor	Dripping from shredder	Lp1 Lp6	LpnS13160 LpnS13161
2	Shredder-Conveyor	Conveyor belt	Lp6 Lp6	LpnS13161 LpnS13162
New York State Department of Health visit (May 17, 2011)				
1	Shredder-Conveyor	Conveyor belt	Lp1 Lp1	LpnS13167 LpnS13168
First site visit (June 1-2, 2011)				
A	Shredder-Outside	Water dripping from gap between water supply pipe and shredder	*feeleii*	Lfe13001
L	Shredder-Exit conveyor	Dripping from shredder onto belt	Lp1 Lp6	LpnS13171 LpnS13170
M	Puddle	Under shredder conveyor belt exit	Lp1	LpnS13169
P	Puddle	Drainage ditch south of shredder	Lp1	LpnS13160
Q	Puddle	Final ferrous pile	Lp1	LpnS13160
R	Picking shed-Conveyor	Conveyor belt	Lp6	LpnS13172
U	Puddle	Under non-ferrous conveyor	Lp1	LpnS13175
W	Puddle	Near non-ferrous conveyor	Lp1 Lp6	LpnS13169 LpnS13174
Y	Puddle	Raw feed pile	Lp1	LpnS13173
Second site visit (September 23, 2011)				
CC	Puddle	Non-ferrous	Lp3	LpnS13191
DD	Puddle	Near shredder conveyor belt exit	Lp1	LpnS13185
M	Puddle	Under shredder conveyor belt exit	Lp1	LpnS13186
L	Shredder-Exit conveyor	Dripping from shredder onto belt	Lp3	LpnS13199
P	Puddle	Drainage ditch south of shredder	Lp1 Lp6	LpnS13187 LpnS13190
O	Pond	Pond	Lp1 Lp3 Lp6 Lp12 Lp sero undetermined	LpnS13196 LpnS16195 LpnS13192 LpnS13194 LpnS13197

*Lp – *L. pneumophila*; the number indicates the serogroup (e.g., Lp1 is *L. pneumophila* serogroup 1).

Table 3. Air sampling results for metals in microgram per cubic meter (µg/m³) collected on June 1-2, 2011

Location	Shredder	Picking shed (inside)	Picking shed (outside)	Near non-ferrous building	West of pond	Outside shredder control room	Grappler crane	Non-ferrous shed	NIOSH REL† (µg/m³)	OSHA PEL‡ (µg/m³)
Aluminum	5.10	3.38	3.31	2.75	(1.08)	2.69	21.25	6.29	10,000 (total) – 5,000 (respirable)	10,000 (total) – 5,000 (respirable)
Antimony	<1.70	<1.30	<1.74	<1.72	<1.30	<1.68	<2.50	<1.66	500	500
Arsenic	<3.40	<2.60	<3.48	<3.44	<2.60	<3.37	<5.00	<3.31	2 (15 minute ceiling), Ca	500
Barium	0.95	0.40	(0.26)	0.57	(0.06)	0.74	2.40	0.71	500	500
Beryllium	<0.01	<0.01	<0.01	<0.01	(0.01)	<0.01	<0.01	<0.01	0.5, Ca	2
Cadmium	<0.05	<0.04	(0.05)	<0.05	<0.04	<0.05	<0.08	(0.05)	Lowest feasible, Ca	5
Calcium	20.41	12.99	10.10	13.40	2.08	13.97	90.00	21.52	-	-
Chromium	<0.17	<0.13	<0.17	<0.17	<0.13	(0.27)	(0.43)	<0.17	500	500
Cobalt	<0.34	<0.26	<0.35	<0.34	<0.26	<0.34	<0.50	<0.34	50	100
Copper	<0.51	<0.39	<0.52	<0.52	<0.39	<0.51	(0.95)	(0.63)	1,000	1,000
Iron	61.22	51.95	33.10	37.80	3.38	38.72	217.50	71.19	5,000	10,000
Lanthanum	<0.34	<0.26	<0.35	<0.34	<0.26	<0.34	<0.50	<0.33	-	-
Lead	<1.19	(1.03)	<1.22	<1.20	<0.91	<1.18	(3.00)	(1.52)	50	50
Lithium	<0.34	<0.26	<0.35	<0.34	<0.26	<0.34	<0.50	<0.33	-	-
Magnesium	4.08	(2.21)	(1.64)	(1.68)	0.78	(2.02)	12.75	3.81	15,000	15,000
Manganese	<3.40	<2.60	<3.48	<3.44	<2.60	<3.37	<5.00	<3.31	1,000	5,000 (ceiling)
Molybdenum	<0.68	<0.52	<0.70	<0.69	<0.52	<0.67	<1.00	<0.66	-	15,000
Nickel	<1.02	<0.78	<1.05	<1.03	<0.78	<1.01	<1.50	<0.99	15, Ca	1,000
Phosphorus	<3.40	<2.60	<3.48	<3.44	<2.60	<3.37	<5.00	<3.31	100	100
Potassium	<10.20	<7.79	<10.45	<10.31	<7.79	<10.10	<15.00	<9.93	-	-
Selenium	<5.10	<3.90	<5.23	<5.15	<3.90	<5.05	<7.50	<4.97	200	-
Silver	<0.17	<0.13	<0.17	<0.17	<0.13	<0.17	<0.25	<0.17	10	10
Strontium	0.19	0.12	(0.07)	(0.09)	(0.03)	(0.12)	0.58	0.20	-	-
Tellurium	<1.53	<1.17	<1.57	<1.55	<1.17	<1.52	<2.25	<1.49	100	100
Thallium	<1.70	<1.30	<1.74	<1.72	<1.30	<1.68	<2.50	<1.66	100	100
Tin	<1.70	<1.30	<1.74	<1.72	<1.30	<1.68	<2.50	<1.66	2,000	2,000
Titanium	(0.15)	(0.09)	(0.16)	<0.10	<0.08	(0.10)	0.55	<0.10	-	-
Vanadium	<0.17	<0.13	<0.17	<0.17	<0.13	<0.17	<0.25	(0.20)	-	-
Yttrium	<0.07	<0.05	<0.07	<0.07	<0.05	<0.07	<0.10	<0.07	1,000	1,000
Zinc	6.97	5.45	3.14	4.30	(0.16)	3.87	18.00	6.95	-	-
Zirconium	<0.12	<0.09	<0.12	<0.12	<0.09	<0.12	<0.18	<0.12	5,000	5,000

†REL: recommended exposure limit; ‡PEL: permissible exposure limit; ( ): values between the limit of detection and the limit of quantification (green); <: value below the limit of detection (purple); Ca: carcinogen.

Figure 1a. Map of facility with *Legionella* sampling locations and results from first visit (June 1-2, 2011).

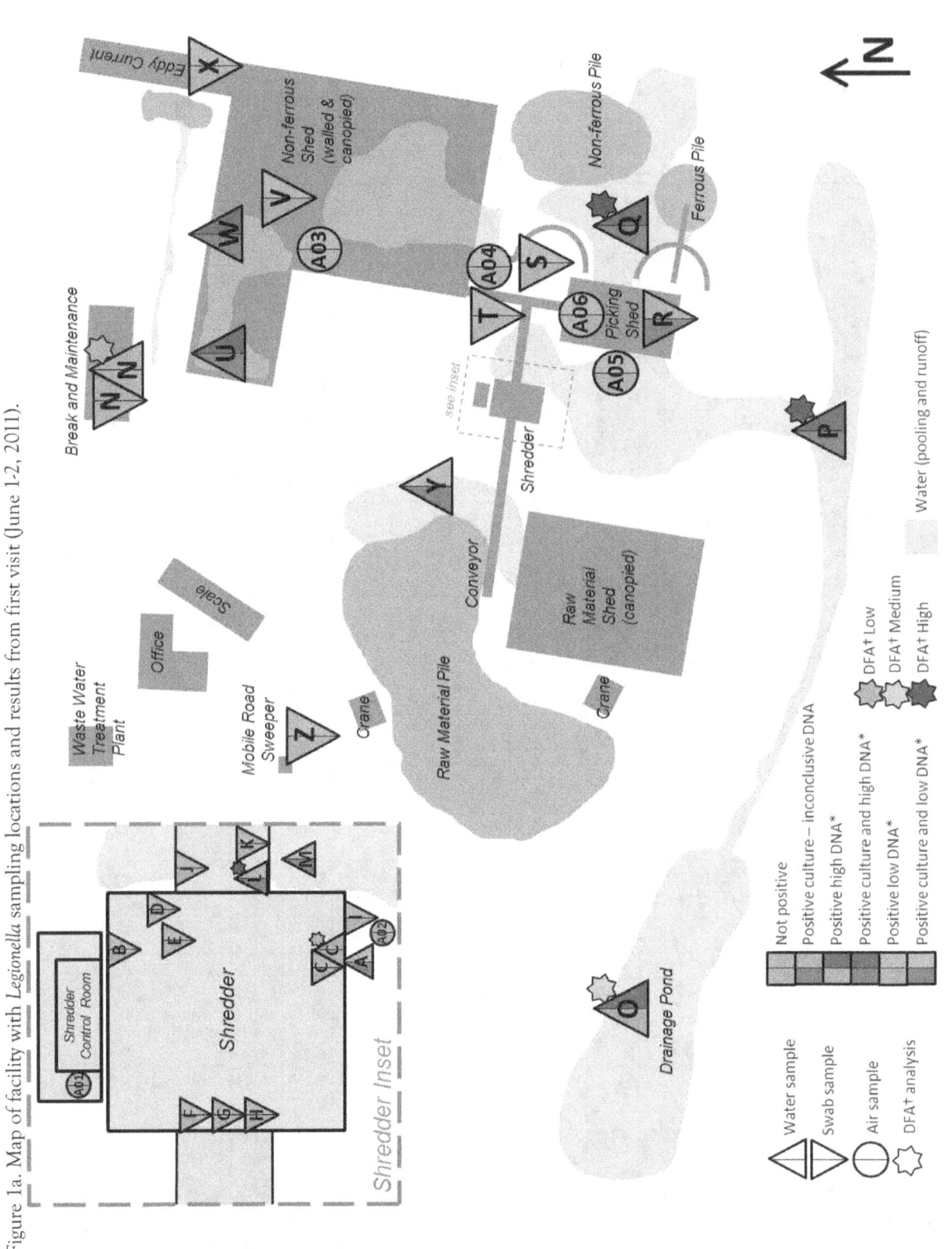

*Samples with high *Legionella* DNA had a lower Ct value while samples with low *Legionella* DNA had a higher Ct value. A Ct value is the cycle in which the sample crossed the PCR threshold. In general, lower Ct values indicate higher numbers of *Legionella* bacteria present while higher Ct values indicate lower numbers of *Legionella* bacteria. †DFA: direct fluorescent antibody.

Figure 1b. Map of facility with *Legionella* sampling locations and results from second visit (September 23, 2011).

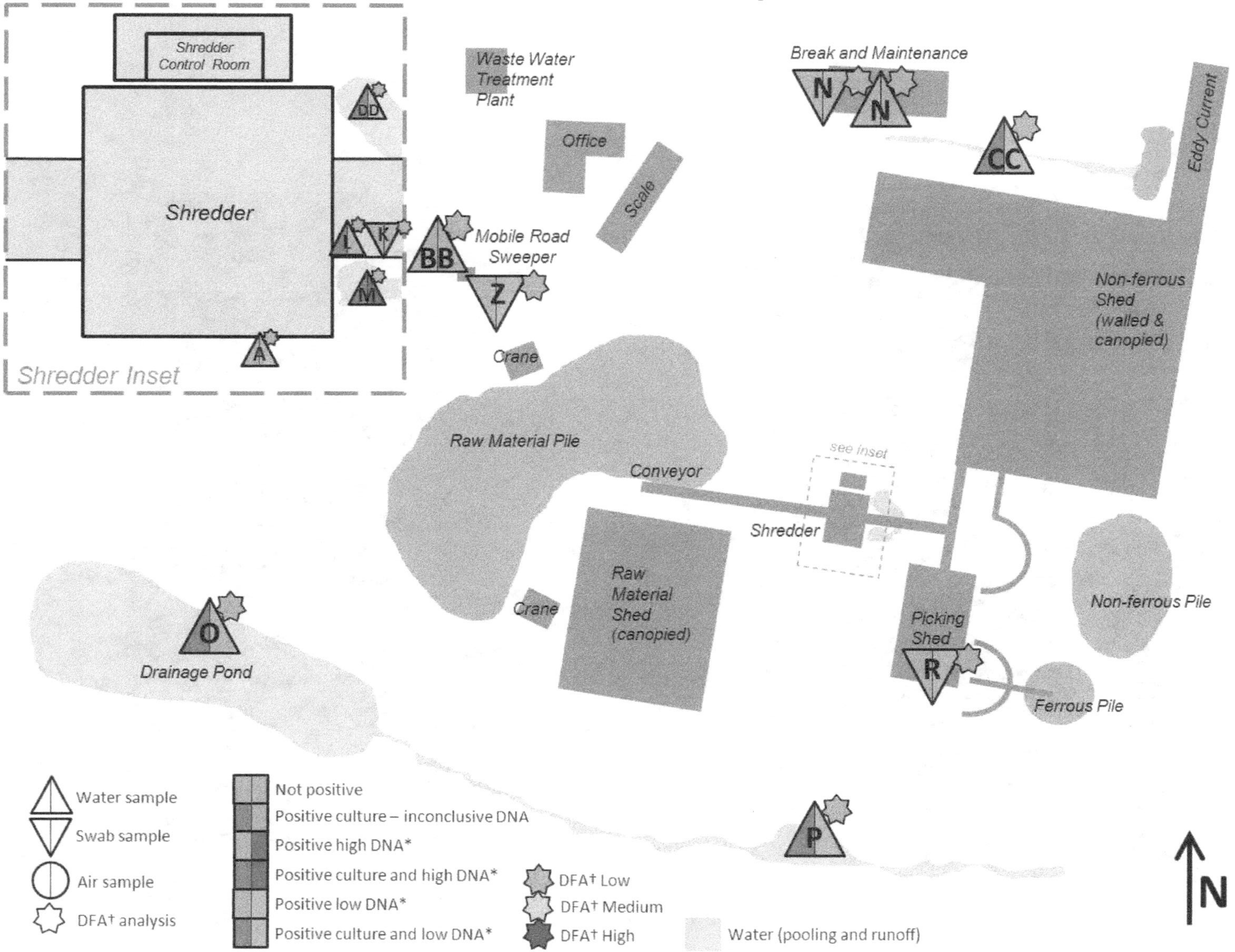

Break and Maintenance

Eddy Current

Non-ferrous Shed (walled & canopied)

Non-ferrous Pile

Ferrous Pile

Picking Shed

see inset

Shredder

Conveyor

Raw Material Shed (canopied)

Raw Material Pile

Crane

Crane

Waste Water Treatment Plant

Office

Scale

Mobile Road Sweeper

Shredder Control Room

Shredder

Shredder Inset

Drainage Pond

N

Water sample ◁

Swab sample ▷

Air sample ○

DFA† analysis ☆

Not positive

Positive culture – inconclusive DNA

Positive high DNA*

Positive culture and high DNA*

Positive low DNA*

Positive culture and low DNA*

DFA† Low

DFA† Medium

DFA† High

Water (pooling and runoff)

*Samples with high *Legionella* DNA had a lower Ct value while samples with low *Legionella* DNA had a higher Ct value. A Ct value is the cycle in which the sample crossed the PCR threshold. In general, lower Ct values indicate higher numbers of *Legionella* bacteria present while higher Ct values indicate lower numbers of *Legionella* bacteria. †DFA: direct fluorescent antibody.

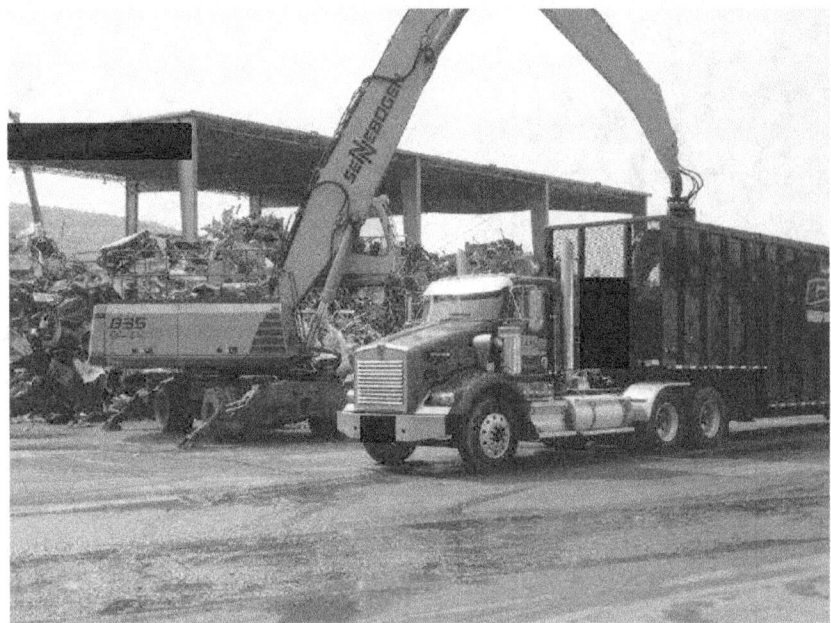

Figure 2. Grappler crane unloading scrap material from truck.

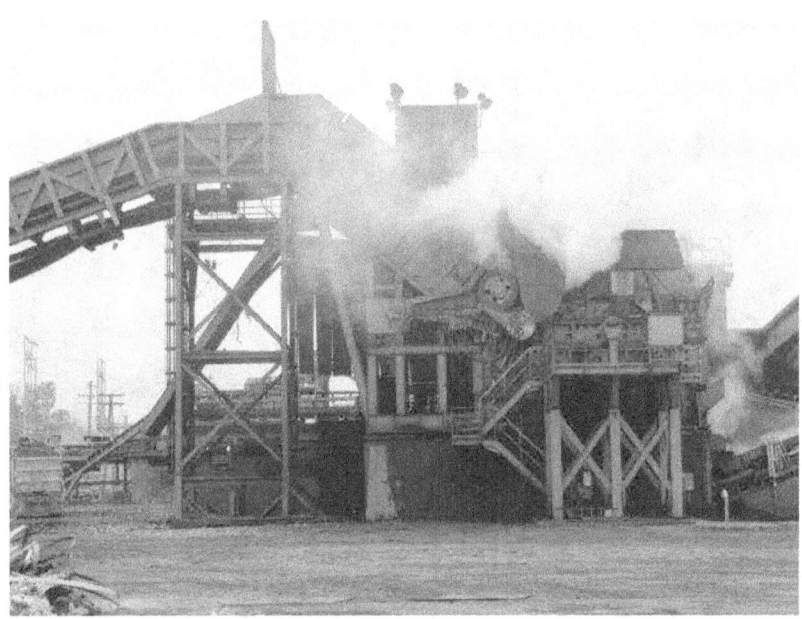

Figure 3. Shredder.

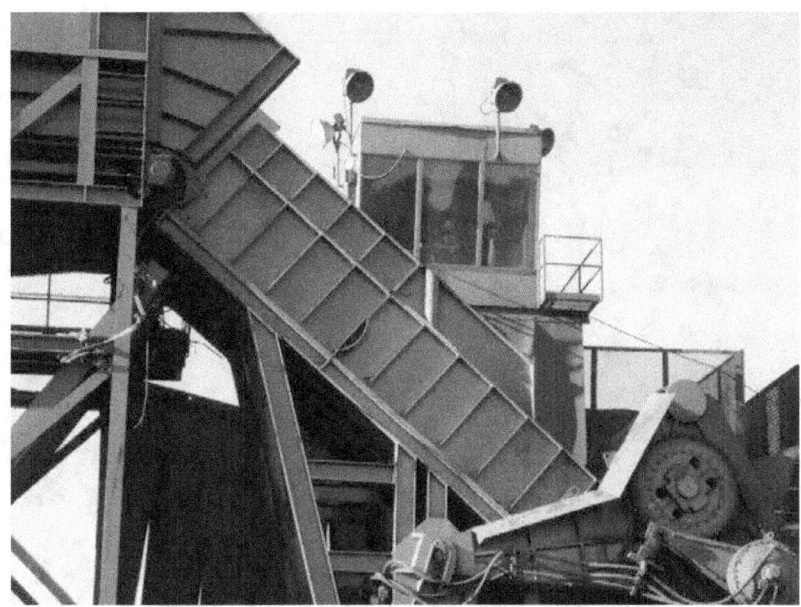

Figure 4. Shredder operator booth.

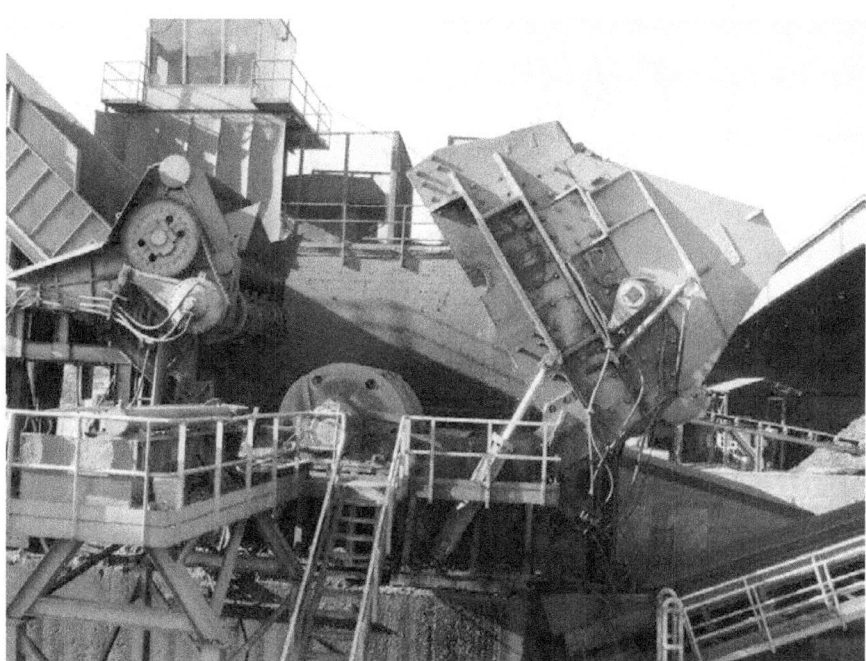

Figure 5. Shredder (top open).

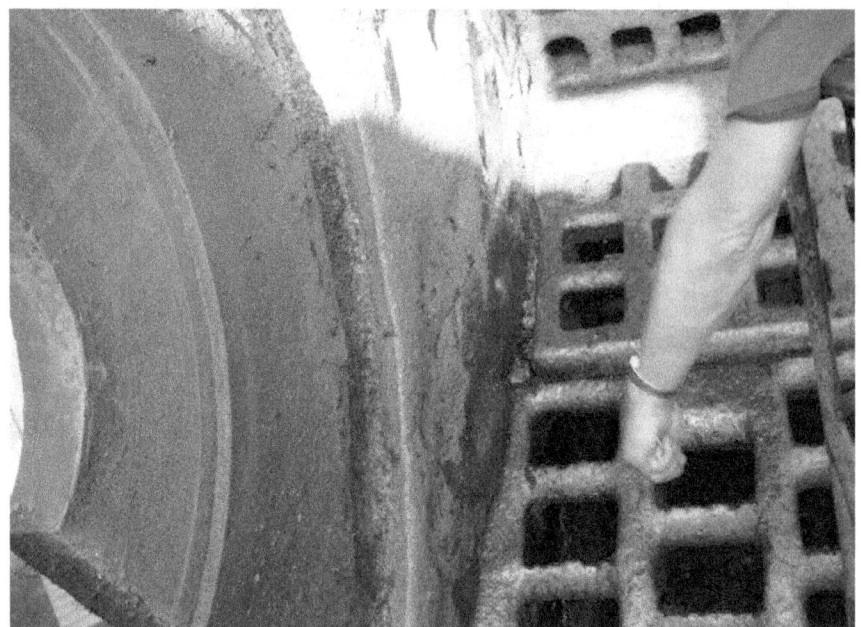

Figure 6. Shredder discharge grate.

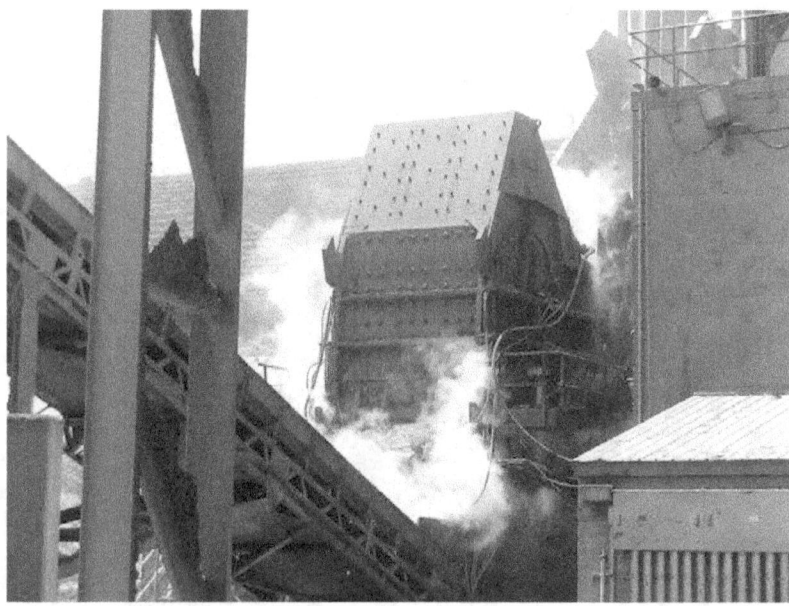

Figure 7. Shredder during operation showing lines that feed water into shredder for cooling.

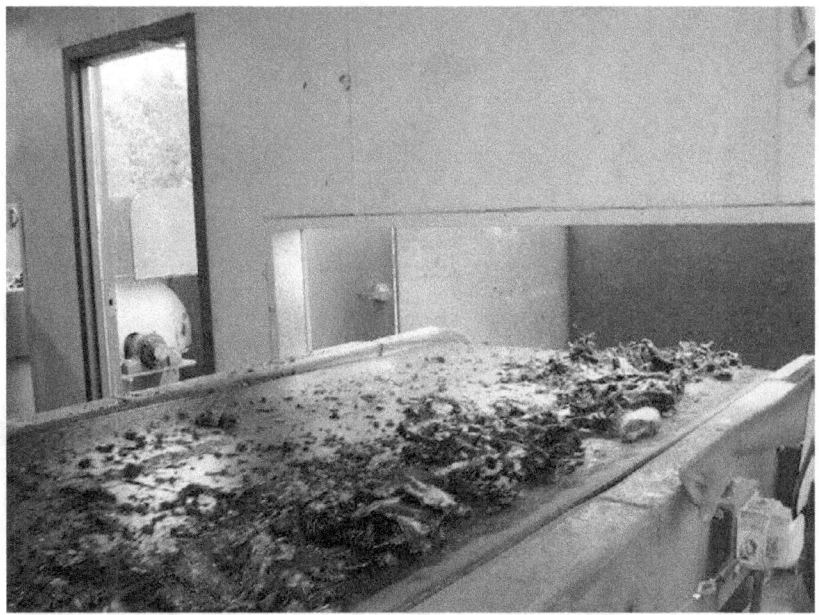

Figure 8. Inside of ferrous metal picking shed where workers remove nonferrous material and copper "meatballs."

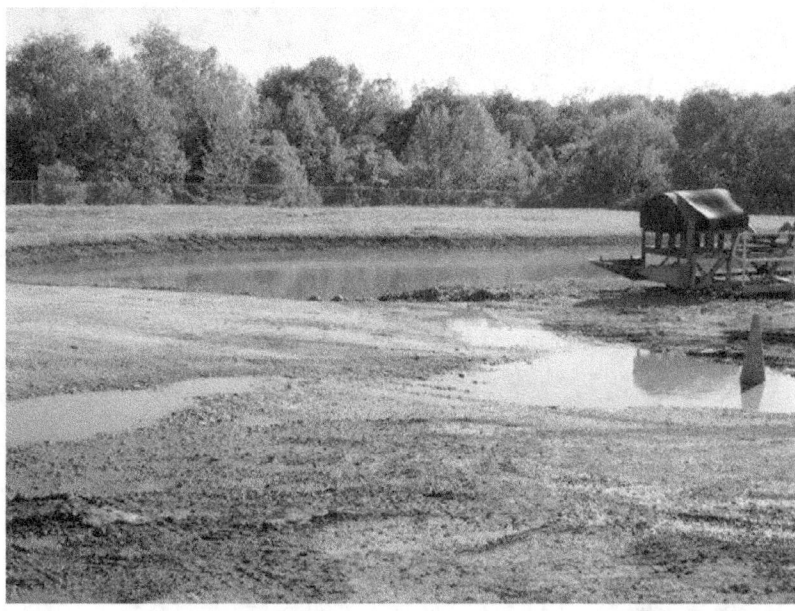

Figure 9. Drainage pond where excess surface water flows by gravity.

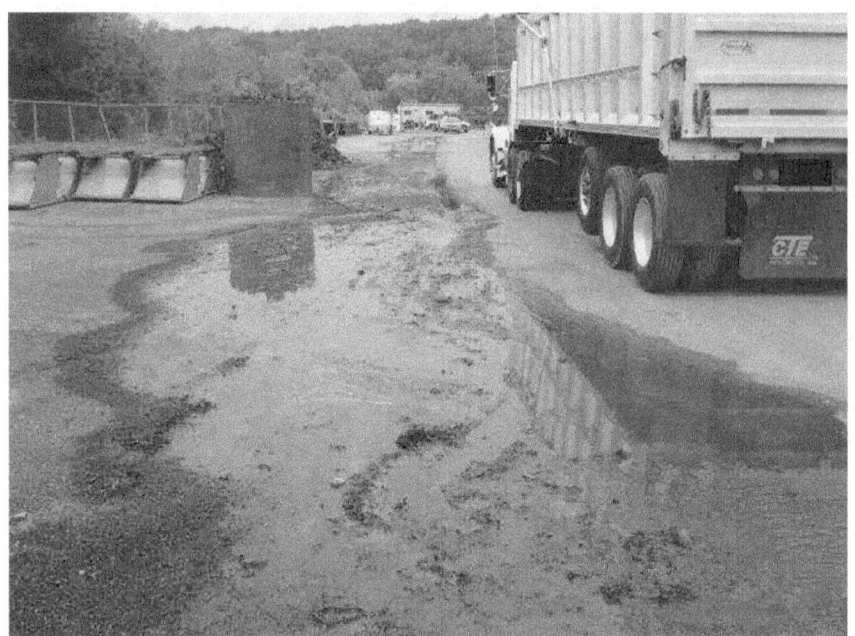

Figure 10. Standing water typical of that found throughout the facility.

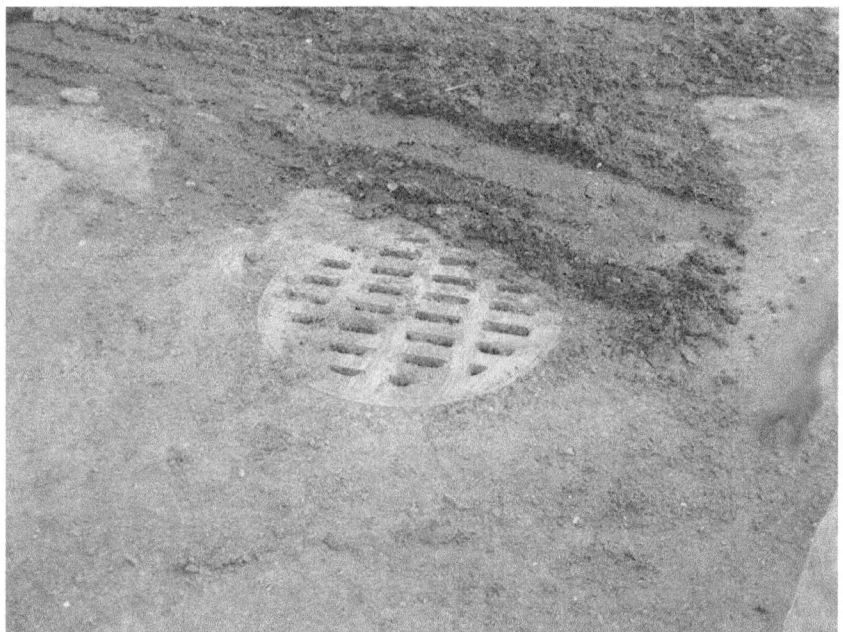

Figure 11. Drain between shredder and picking shed.

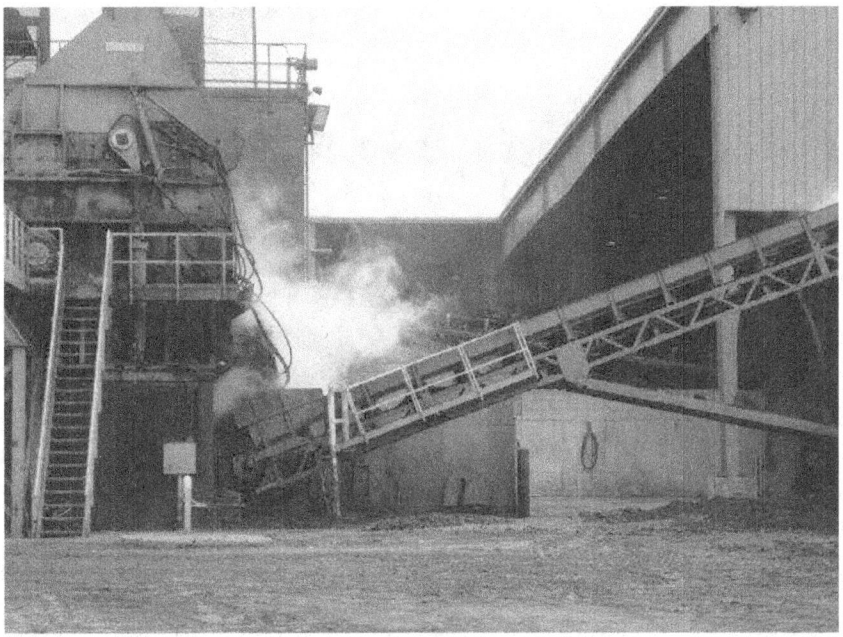

Figure 12. Steam emitted from shredder during operation.

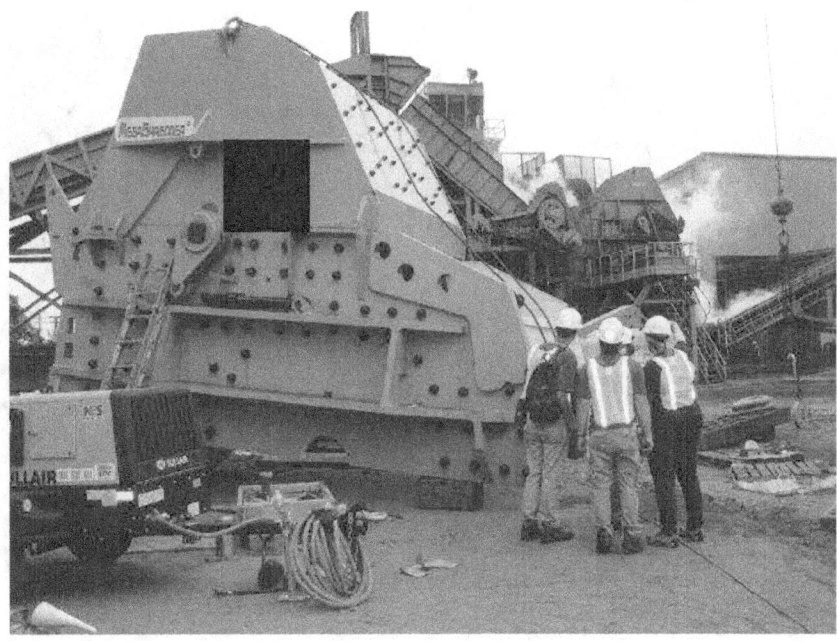

Figure 13. New shredder being prepared for installation.

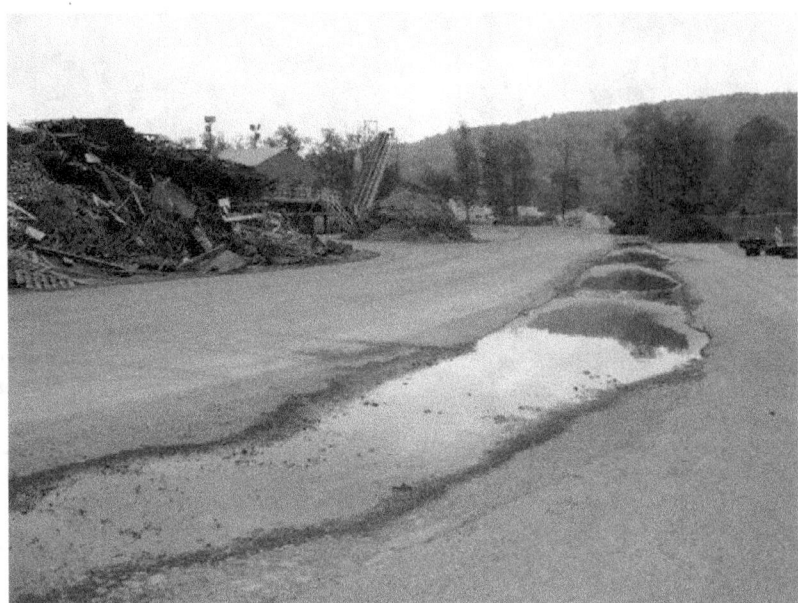

Figure 14. Pool of standing water on the south side of the facility (looking east).

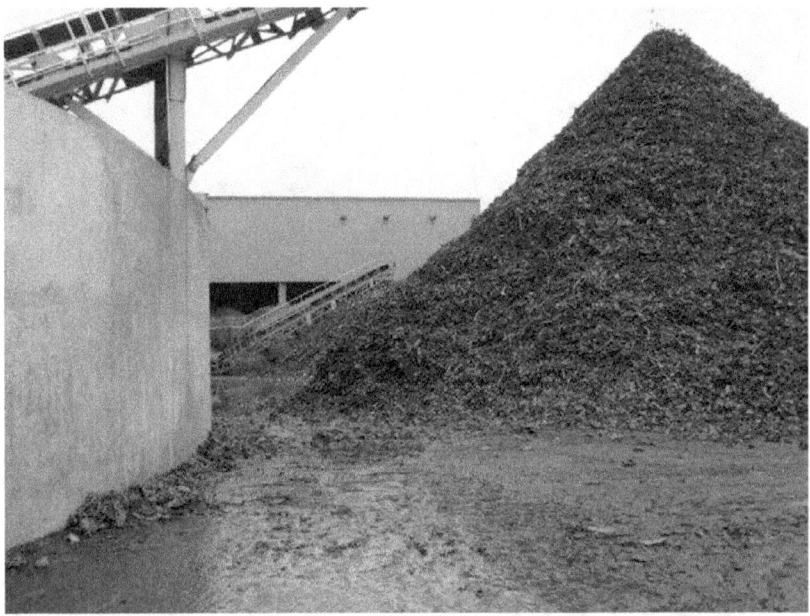

Figure 15. Conveyor (foreground) that exits picking shed near ferrous pile. Non-ferrous conveyor, pile, and shed are in the background. Standing water is present in the foreground and between the two piles.

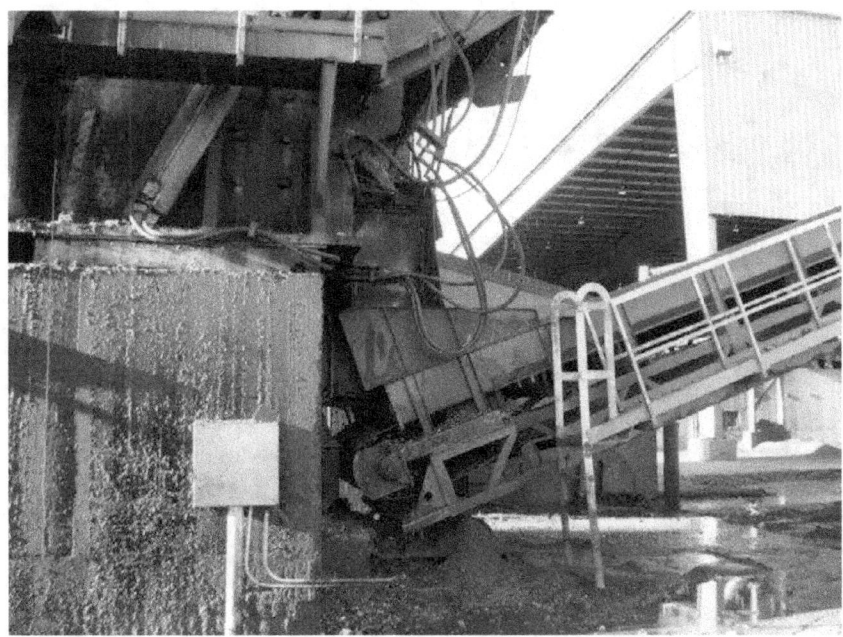

Figure 16. Conveyor at the exit of the shredder. Standing water is present near the shredder, under the conveyor, and in the background of the photograph. Water drips from the shredder onto the belt and from the belt onto the ground.

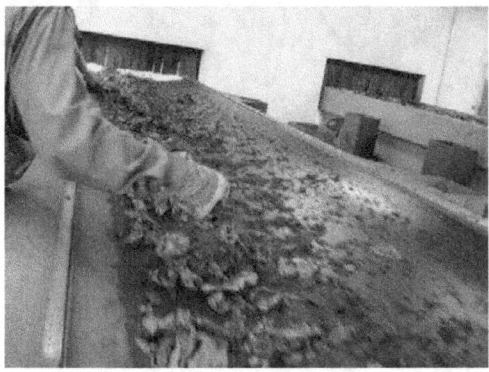

(a)

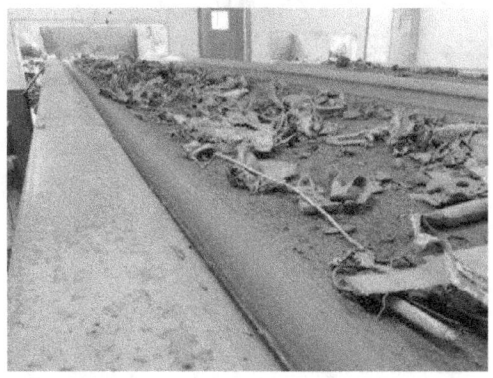

(b)

Figure 17. Conveyor belt in picking shed with (a) wet material during first visit and (b) drier material during second visit.

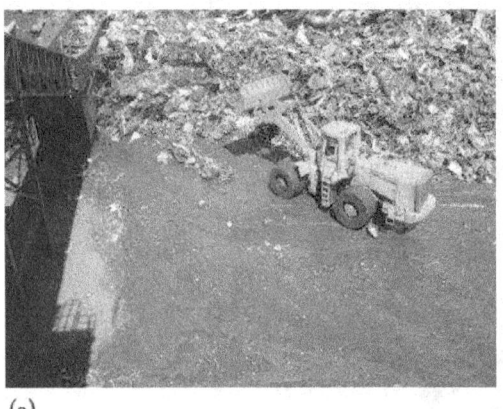
(a)

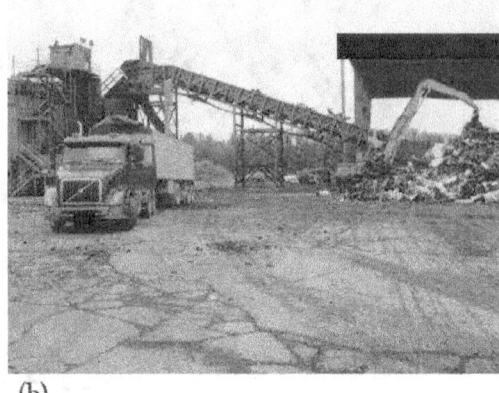
(b)

Figure 18. (a) Loader driving through a large pool of water while moving scrap from the raw feed pile to the shredder feed conveyor during first visit. (b) Area under conveyor as in Figure (a), but taken from a different angle during the second visit. Green crane is in same position as yellow loader in Figure (a). Less water is evident.

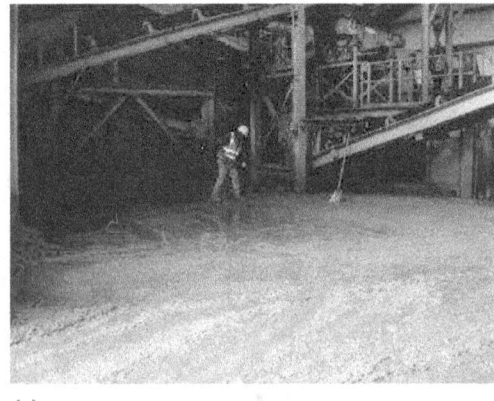
(a)

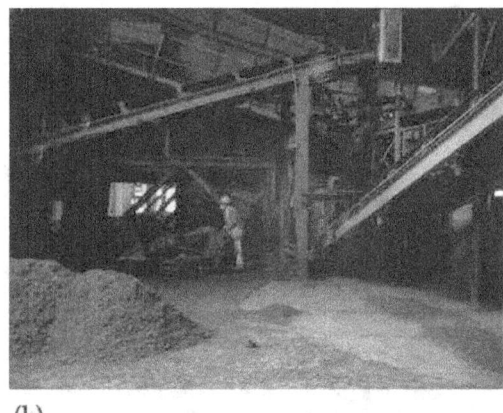
(b)

Figure 19. Worker removing debris from under a conveyor in the non-ferrous shed during (a) first visit and (b) second visit. Pooled water eliminated between visits.

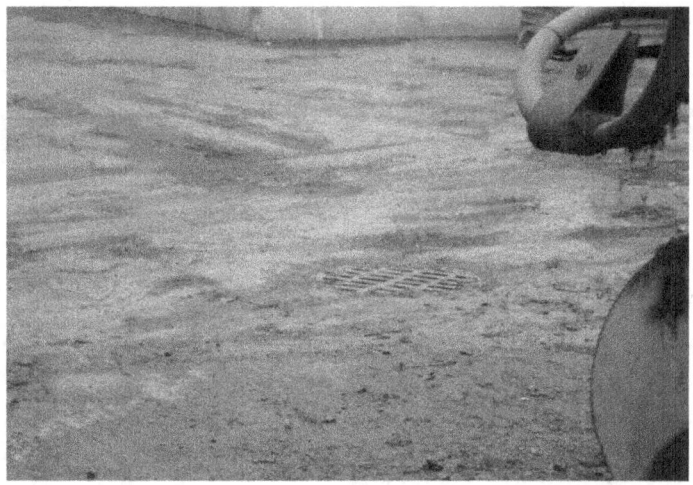

Figure 20. A drain grate that was uncovered during re-grading operations.

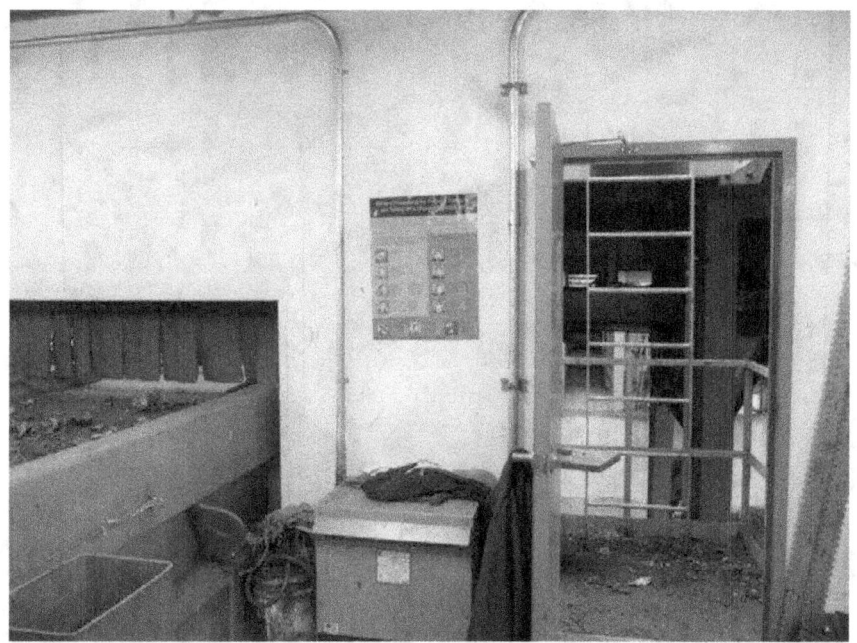

Figure 21. NIOSH poster in picking shed showing how to put on and take off an N-95 respirator.

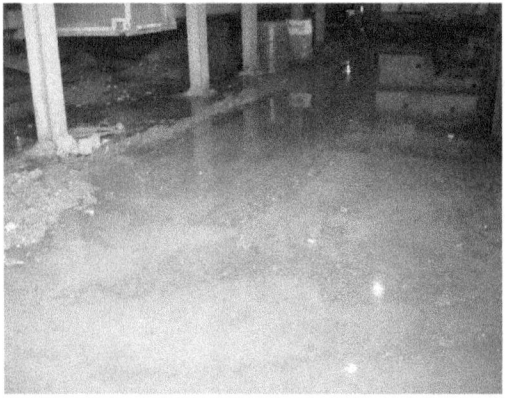
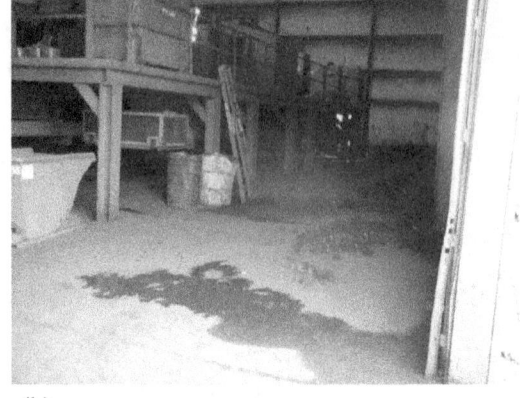

(a)   (b)

Figure 22. (a) Pool of standing water in the non-ferrous shed during the first visit. (b) Same area during second visit showing the reduction in water.

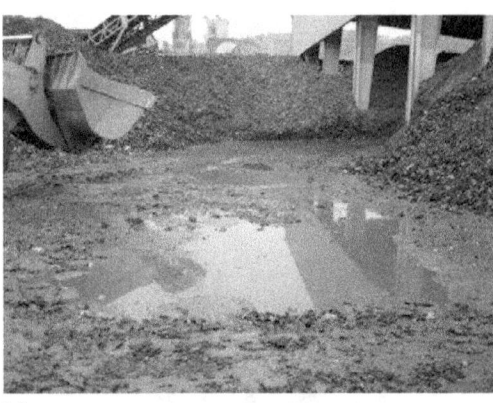
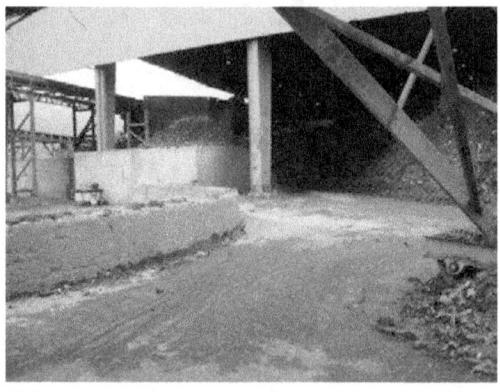

(a)   (b)

Figure 23. (a) Pool of standing water near the non-ferrous shed during the first visit. (b) Same area during second visit showing the reduction in water.

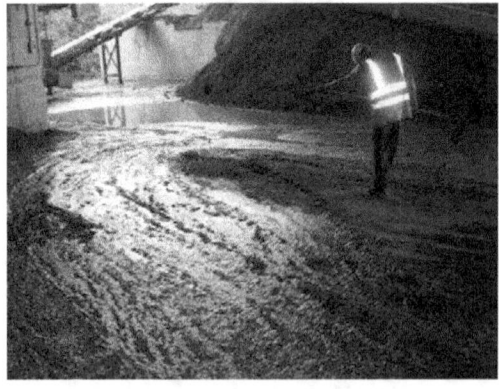
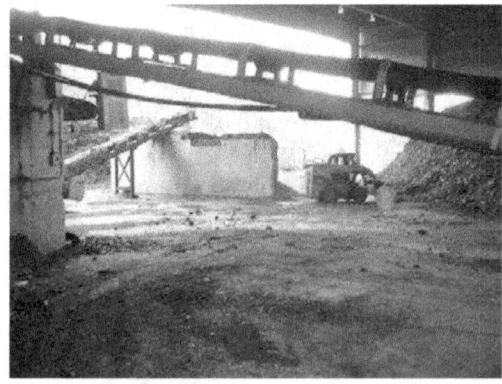

(a)   (b)

Figure 24. (a) Worker shoveling debris in non-ferrous shed during first visit. Standing water and tracks from mobile equipment can be seen. (b) Same area during second visit showing the reduction in water.

APPENDIX A: APPENDIX A OF OSHA RESPIRATORY PROTECTION STANDARD

Appendix A: Appendix A to § 1910.134: Fit Testing Procedures (Mandatory)

Part I. OSHA-Accepted Fit Test Protocols

A. Fit Testing Procedures - General Requirements

The employer shall conduct fit testing using the following procedures. The requirements in this appendix apply to all OSHA-accepted fit test methods, both QLFT and QNFT.

1. The test subject shall be allowed to pick the most acceptable respirator from a sufficient number of respirator models and sizes so that the respirator is acceptable to, and correctly fits, the user.

2. Prior to the selection process, the test subject shall be shown how to put on a respirator, how it should be positioned on the face, how to set strap tension and how to determine an acceptable fit. A mirror shall be available to assist the subject in evaluating the fit and positioning of the respirator. This instruction may not constitute the subject's formal training on respirator use, because it is only a review.

3. The test subject shall be informed that he/she is being asked to select the respirator that provides the most acceptable fit. Each respirator represents a different size and shape, and if fitted and used properly, will provide adequate protection.

4. The test subject shall be instructed to hold each chosen facepiece up to the face and eliminate those that obviously do not give an acceptable fit.

5. The more acceptable facepieces are noted in case the one selected proves unacceptable; the most comfortable mask is donned and worn at least five minutes to assess comfort. Assistance in assessing comfort can be given by discussing the points in the following item A.6. If the test subject is not familiar with using a particular respirator, the test subject shall be directed to don the mask several times and to adjust the straps each time to become adept at setting proper tension on the straps.

6. Assessment of comfort shall include a review of the following points with the test subject and allowing the test subject adequate time to determine the comfort of the respirator:

   (a) Position of the mask on the nose

   (b) Room for eye protection

   (c) Room to talk

   (d) Position of mask on face and cheeks

7. The following criteria shall be used to help determine the adequacy of the respirator fit:

   (a) Chin properly placed;

   (b) Adequate strap tension, not overly tightened;

(c) Fit across nose bridge;

(d) Respirator of proper size to span distance from nose to chin;

(e) Tendency of respirator to slip;

(f) Self-observation in mirror to evaluate fit and respirator position.

8. The test subject shall conduct a user seal check, either the negative and positive pressure seal checks described in Appendix B-1 of this section or those recommended by the respirator manufacturer which provide equivalent protection to the procedures in Appendix B-1. Before conducting the negative and positive pressure checks, the subject shall be told to seat the mask on the face by moving the head from side-to-side and up and down slowly while taking in a few slow deep breaths. Another facepiece shall be selected and retested if the test subject fails the user seal check tests.

9. The test shall not be conducted if there is any hair growth between the skin and the facepiece sealing surface, such as stubble beard growth, beard, mustache or sideburns which cross the respirator sealing surface. Any type of apparel which interferes with a satisfactory fit shall be altered or removed.

10. If a test subject exhibits difficulty in breathing during the tests, she or he shall be referred to a physician or other licensed health care professional, as appropriate, to determine whether the test subject can wear a respirator while performing her or his duties.

11. If the employee finds the fit of the respirator unacceptable, the test subject shall be given the opportunity to select a different respirator and to be retested.

12. Exercise regimen. Prior to the commencement of the fit test, the test subject shall be given a description of the fit test and the test subject's responsibilities during the test procedure. The description of the process shall include a description of the test exercises that the subject will be performing. The respirator to be tested shall be worn for at least 5 minutes before the start of the fit test.

13. The fit test shall be performed while the test subject is wearing any applicable safety equipment that may be worn during actual respirator use which could interfere with respirator fit.

14. Test Exercises.

(a) Employers must perform the following test exercises for all fit testing methods prescribed in this appendix, except for the CNP quantitative fit testing protocol and the CNP REDON quantitative fit testing protocol. For these two protocols, employers must ensure that the test subjects (i.e., employees) perform the exercise procedure specified in Part I.C.4(b) of this appendix for the CNP quantitative fit testing protocol, or the exercise procedure described in Part I.C.5(b) of this appendix for the CNP REDON quantitative fit-testing protocol. For the remaining fit testing methods, employers must ensure that employees perform the test exercises in the appropriate test environment in the following manner:

(1) Normal breathing. In a normal standing position, without talking, the subject shall

breathe normally.

(2) Deep breathing. In a normal standing position, the subject shall breathe slowly and deeply, taking caution so as not to hyperventilate.

(3) Turning head side to side. Standing in place, the subject shall slowly turn his/her head from side to side between the extreme positions on each side. The head shall be held at each extreme momentarily so the subject can inhale at each side.

(4) Moving head up and down. Standing in place, the subject shall slowly move his/her head up and down. The subject shall be instructed to inhale in the up position (i.e., when looking toward the ceiling).

(5) Talking. The subject shall talk out loud slowly and loud enough so as to be heard clearly by the test conductor. The subject can read from a prepared text such as the Rainbow Passage, count backward from 100, or recite a memorized poem or song.

Rainbow Passage

When the sunlight strikes raindrops in the air, they act like a prism and form a rainbow. The rainbow is a division of white light into many beautiful colors. These take the shape of a long round arch, with its path high above, and its two ends apparently beyond the horizon. There is, according to legend, a boiling pot of gold at one end. People look, but no one ever finds it. When a man looks for something beyond reach, his friends say he is looking for the pot of gold at the end of the rainbow.

(6) Grimace. The test subject shall grimace by smiling or frowning. (This applies only to QNFT testing; it is not performed for QLFT)

(7) Bending over. The test subject shall bend at the waist as if he/she were to touch his/her toes. Jogging in place shall be substituted for this exercise in those test environments such as shroud type QNFT or QLFT units that do not permit bending over at the waist.

(8) Normal breathing. Same as exercise (1).

(b) Each test exercise shall be performed for one minute except for the grimace exercise which shall be performed for 15 seconds. The test subject shall be questioned by the test conductor regarding the comfort of the respirator upon completion of the protocol. If it has become unacceptable, another model of respirator shall be tried. The respirator shall not be adjusted once the fit test exercises begin. Any adjustment voids the test, and the fit test must be repeated.

B. Qualitative Fit Test (QLFT) Protocols

1. General

(a) The employer shall ensure that persons administering QLFT are able to prepare test solutions, calibrate equipment and perform tests properly, recognize invalid tests, and ensure that test equipment is in proper working order.

(b) The employer shall ensure that QLFT equipment is kept clean and well maintained so as to operate within the parameters for which it was designed.

2. Isoamyl Acetate Protocol

Note: This protocol is not appropriate to use for the fit testing of particulate respirators. If used to fit test particulate respirators, the respirator must be equipped with an organic vapor filter.

(a) Odor Threshold Screening

Odor threshold screening, performed without wearing a respirator, is intended to determine if the individual tested can detect the odor of isoamyl acetate at low levels.

(1) Three 1 liter glass jars with metal lids are required.

(2) Odor-free water (e.g., distilled or spring water) at approximately 25 deg. C (77 deg. F) shall be used for the solutions.

(3) The isoamyl acetate (IAA) (also known at isopentyl acetate) stock solution is prepared by adding 1 ml of pure IAA to 800 ml of odor-free water in a 1 liter jar, closing the lid and shaking for 30 seconds. A new solution shall be prepared at least weekly.

(4) The screening test shall be conducted in a room separate from the room used for actual fit testing. The two rooms shall be well-ventilated to prevent the odor of IAA from becoming evident in the general room air where testing takes place.

(5) The odor test solution is prepared in a second jar by placing 0.4 ml of the stock solution into 500 ml of odor-free water using a clean dropper or pipette. The solution shall be shaken for 30 seconds and allowed to stand for two to three minutes so that the IAA concentration above the liquid may reach equilibrium. This solution shall be used for only one day.

(6) A test blank shall be prepared in a third jar by adding 500 cc of odor-free water.

(7) The odor test and test blank jar lids shall be labeled (e.g., 1 and 2) for jar identification. Labels shall be placed on the lids so that they can be peeled off periodically and switched to maintain the integrity of the test.

(8) The following instruction shall be typed on a card and placed on the table in front of the two test jars (i.e., 1 and 2): "The purpose of this test is to determine if you can smell banana oil at a low concentration. The two bottles in front of you contain water. One of these bottles also contains a small amount of banana oil. Be sure the covers are on tight, then shake each bottle for two seconds. Unscrew the lid of each bottle, one at a time,

and sniff at the mouth of the bottle. Indicate to the test conductor which bottle contains banana oil."

(9) The mixtures used in the IAA odor detection test shall be prepared in an area separate from where the test is performed, in order to prevent olfactory fatigue in the subject.

(10) If the test subject is unable to correctly identify the jar containing the odor test solution, the IAA qualitative fit test shall not be performed.

(11) If the test subject correctly identifies the jar containing the odor test solution, the test subject may proceed to respirator selection and fit testing.

(b) Isoamyl Acetate Fit Test

(1) The fit test chamber shall be a clear 55-gallon drum liner suspended inverted over a 2-foot diameter frame so that the top of the chamber is about 6 inches above the test subject's head. If no drum liner is available, a similar chamber shall be constructed using plastic sheeting. The inside top center of the chamber shall have a small hook attached.

(2) Each respirator used for the fitting and fit testing shall be equipped with organic vapor cartridges or offer protection against organic vapors.

(3) After selecting, donning, and properly adjusting a respirator, the test subject shall wear it to the fit testing room. This room shall be separate from the room used for odor threshold screening and respirator selection, and shall be well-ventilated, as by an exhaust fan or lab hood, to prevent general room contamination.

(4) A copy of the test exercises and any prepared text from which the subject is to read shall be taped to the inside of the test chamber.

(5) Upon entering the test chamber, the test subject shall be given a 6-inch by 5-inch piece of paper towel, or other porous, absorbent, single-ply material, folded in half and wetted with 0.75 ml of pure IAA. The test subject shall hang the wet towel on the hook at the top of the chamber. An IAA test swab or ampule may be substituted for the IAA wetted paper towel provided it has been demonstrated that the alternative IAA source will generate an IAA test atmosphere with a concentration equivalent to that generated by the paper towel method.

(6) Allow two minutes for the IAA test concentration to stabilize before starting the fit test exercises. This would be an appropriate time to talk with the test subject; to explain the fit test, the importance of his/her cooperation, and the purpose for the test exercises; or to demonstrate some of the exercises.

(7) If at any time during the test, the subject detects the banana-like odor of IAA, the test is failed. The subject shall quickly exit from the test chamber and leave the test area to avoid olfactory fatigue.

(8) If the test is failed, the subject shall return to the selection room and remove the respirator. The test subject shall repeat the odor sensitivity test, select and put on another respirator, return to the test area and again begin the fit test procedure described in (b) (1) through (7) above. The process continues until a respirator that fits well has been found. Should the odor sensitivity test be failed, the subject shall wait at least 5 minutes before retesting. Odor sensitivity will usually have returned by this time.

(9) If the subject passes the test, the efficiency of the test procedure shall be demonstrated by having the subject break the respirator face seal and take a breath before exiting the chamber.

(10) When the test subject leaves the chamber, the subject shall remove the saturated towel and return it to the person conducting the test, so that there is no significant IAA concentration buildup in the chamber during subsequent tests. The used towels shall be kept in a self-sealing plastic bag to keep the test area from being contaminated.

3. Saccharin Solution Aerosol Protocol

The entire screening and testing procedure shall be explained to the test subject prior to the conduct of the screening test.

(a) Taste threshold screening. The saccharin taste threshold screening, performed without wearing a respirator, is intended to determine whether the individual being tested can detect the taste of saccharin.

(1) During threshold screening as well as during fit testing, subjects shall wear an enclosure about the head and shoulders that is approximately 12 inches in diameter by 14 inches tall with at least the front portion clear and that allows free movements of the head when a respirator is worn. An enclosure substantially similar to the 3M hood assembly, parts # FT 14 and # FT 15 combined, is adequate.

(2) The test enclosure shall have a 3/4-inch (1 9 cm) hole in front of the test subject's nose and mouth area to accommodate the nebulizer nozzle.

(3) The test subject shall don the test enclosure. Throughout the threshold screening test, the test subject shall breathe through his/her slightly open mouth with tongue extended. The subject is instructed to report when he/she detects a sweet taste.

(4) Using a DeVilbiss Model 40 Inhalation Medication Nebulizer or equivalent, the test conductor shall spray the threshold check solution into the enclosure. The nozzle is directed away from the nose and mouth of the person. This nebulizer shall be clearly marked to distinguish it from the fit test solution nebulizer.

(5) The threshold check solution is prepared by dissolving 0.83 gram of sodium saccharin USP in 100 ml of warm water. It can be prepared by putting 1 ml of the fit test solution (see (b)(5) below) in 100 ml of distilled water.

(6) To produce the aerosol, the nebulizer bulb is firmly squeezed so that it collapses completely, then released and allowed to fully expand.

(7) Ten squeezes are repeated rapidly and then the test subject is asked whether the saccharin can be tasted. If the test subject reports tasting the sweet taste during the ten squeezes, the screening test is completed. The taste threshold is noted as ten regardless of the number of squeezes actually completed.

(8) If the first response is negative, ten more squeezes are repeated rapidly and the test subject is again asked whether the saccharin is tasted. If the test subject reports tasting the sweet taste during the second ten squeezes, the screening test is completed. The taste threshold is noted as twenty regardless of the number of squeezes actually completed.

(9) If the second response is negative, ten more squeezes are repeated rapidly and the test subject is again asked whether the saccharin is tasted. If the test subject reports tasting the sweet taste during the third set of ten squeezes, the screening test is completed. The taste threshold is noted as thirty regardless of the number of squeezes actually completed.

(10) The test conductor will take note of the number of squeezes required to solicit a taste response.

(11) If the saccharin is not tasted after 30 squeezes (step 10), the test subject is unable to taste saccharin and may not perform the saccharin fit test.

Note to paragraph 3. (a): If the test subject eats or drinks something sweet before the screening test, he/she may be unable to taste the weak saccharin solution.

(12) If a taste response is elicited, the test subject shall be asked to take note of the taste for reference in the fit test.

(13) Correct use of the nebulizer means that approximately 1 ml of liquid is used at a time in the nebulizer body.

(14) The nebulizer shall be thoroughly rinsed in water, shaken dry, and refilled at least each morning and afternoon or at least every four hours.

(b) Saccharin solution aerosol fit test procedure.

(1) The test subject may not eat, drink (except plain water), smoke, or chew gum for 15 minutes before the test.

(2) The fit test uses the same enclosure described in 3. (a) above.

(3) The test subject shall don the enclosure while wearing the respirator selected in section I. A. of this appendix. The respirator shall be properly adjusted and equipped with a particulate filter(s).

(4) A second DeVilbiss Model 40 Inhalation Medication Nebulizer or equivalent is used to spray the fit test solution into the enclosure. This nebulizer shall be clearly marked to distinguish it from the screening test solution nebulizer.

(5) The fit test solution is prepared by adding 83 grams of sodium saccharin to 100 ml of warm water.

(6) As before, the test subject shall breathe through the slightly open mouth with tongue extended, and report if he/she tastes the sweet taste of saccharin.

(7) The nebulizer is inserted into the hole in the front of the enclosure and an initial concentration of saccharin fit test solution is sprayed into the enclosure using the same number of squeezes (either 10, 20 or 30 squeezes) based on the number of squeezes required to elicit a taste response as noted during the screening test. A minimum of 10 squeezes is required.

(8) After generating the aerosol, the test subject shall be instructed to perform the exercises in section I. A. 14. of this appendix.

(9) Every 30 seconds the aerosol concentration shall be replenished using one half the original number of squeezes used initially (e.g., 5, 10 or 15).

(10) The test subject shall indicate to the test conductor if at any time during the fit test the taste of saccharin is detected. If the test subject does not report tasting the saccharin, the test is passed.

(11) If the taste of saccharin is detected, the fit is deemed unsatisfactory and the test is failed. A different respirator shall be tried and the entire test procedure is repeated (taste threshold screening and fit testing).

(12) Since the nebulizer has a tendency to clog during use, the test operator must make periodic checks of the nebulizer to ensure that it is not clogged. If clogging is found at the end of the test session, the test is invalid.

4. Bitrex™ (Denatonium Benzoate) Solution Aerosol Qualitative Fit Test Protocol

The Bitrex™ (Denatonium benzoate) solution aerosol QLFT protocol uses the published saccharin test protocol because that protocol is widely accepted. Bitrex is routinely used as a taste aversion agent in household liquids which children should not be drinking and is endorsed by the American Medical Association, the National Safety Council, and the American Association of Poison Control Centers. The entire screening and testing procedure shall be explained to the test subject prior to the conduct of the screening test.

(a) Taste Threshold Screening.

The Bitrex taste threshold screening, performed without wearing a respirator, is intended to determine whether the individual being tested can detect the taste of Bitrex.

(1) During threshold screening as well as during fit testing, subjects shall wear an enclosure about the head and shoulders that is approximately 12 inches (30.5 cm) in diameter by 14 inches (35.6 cm) tall. The front portion of the enclosure shall be clear from the respirator and allow free movement of the head when a respirator is worn. An enclosure substantially similar to the 3M hood assembly, parts # FT 14 and # FT 15 combined, is adequate.

(2) The test enclosure shall have a \3/4\ inch (1.9 cm) hole in front of the test subject's nose and mouth area to accommodate the nebulizer nozzle.

(3) The test subject shall don the test enclosure. Throughout the threshold screening test, the test subject shall breathe through his or her slightly open mouth with tongue extended. The subject is instructed to report when he/she detects a bitter taste

(4) Using a DeVilbiss Model 40 Inhalation Medication Nebulizer or equivalent, the test conductor shall spray the Threshold Check Solution into the enclosure. This Nebulizer shall be clearly marked to distinguish it from the fit test solution nebulizer.

(5) The Threshold Check Solution is prepared by adding 13.5 milligrams of Bitrex to 100 ml of 5% salt (NaCl) solution in distilled water.

(6) To produce the aerosol, the nebulizer bulb is firmly squeezed so that the bulb collapses completely, and is then released and allowed to fully expand.

(7) An initial ten squeezes are repeated rapidly and then the test subject is asked whether the Bitrex can be tasted. If the test subject reports tasting the bitter taste during the ten squeezes, the screening test is completed. The taste threshold is noted as ten regardless of the number of squeezes actually completed.

(8) If the first response is negative, ten more squeezes are repeated rapidly and the test subject is again asked whether the Bitrex is tasted. If the test subject reports tasting the bitter taste during the second ten squeezes, the screening test is completed. The taste threshold is noted as twenty regardless of the number of squeezes actually completed.

(9) If the second response is negative, ten more squeezes are repeated rapidly and the test subject is again asked whether the Bitrex is tasted. If the test subject reports tasting the bitter taste during the third set of ten squeezes, the screening test is completed. The taste threshold is noted as thirty regardless of the number of squeezes actually completed.

(10) The test conductor will take note of the number of squeezes required to solicit a taste response.

(11) If the Bitrex is not tasted after 30 squeezes (step 10), the test subject is unable to taste

Bitrex and may not perform the Bitrex fit test.

(12) If a taste response is elicited, the test subject shall be asked to take note of the taste for reference in the fit test.

(13) Correct use of the nebulizer means that approximately 1 ml of liquid is used at a time in the nebulizer body.

(14) The nebulizer shall be thoroughly rinsed in water, shaken to dry, and refilled at least each morning and afternoon or at least every four hours.

(b) Bitrex Solution Aerosol Fit Test Procedure.

(1) The test subject may not eat, drink (except plain water), smoke, or chew gum for 15 minutes before the test.

(2) The fit test uses the same enclosure as that described in 4. (a) above.

(3) The test subject shall don the enclosure while wearing the respirator selected according to section I. A. of this appendix. The respirator shall be properly adjusted and equipped with any type particulate filter(s).

(4) A second DeVilbiss Model 40 Inhalation Medication Nebulizer or equivalent is used to spray the fit test solution into the enclosure. This nebulizer shall be clearly marked to distinguish it from the screening test solution nebulizer.

(5) The fit test solution is prepared by adding 337 5 mg of Bitrex to 200 ml of a 5% salt (NaCl) solution in warm water.

(6) As before, the test subject shall breathe through his or her slightly open mouth with tongue extended, and be instructed to report if he/she tastes the bitter taste of Bitrex.

(7) The nebulizer is inserted into the hole in the front of the enclosure and an initial concentration of the fit test solution is sprayed into the enclosure using the same number of squeezes (either 10, 20 or 30 squeezes) based on the number of squeezes required to elicit a taste response as noted during the screening test.

(8) After generating the aerosol, the test subject shall be instructed to perform the exercises in section I. A. 14. of this appendix.

(9) Every 30 seconds the aerosol concentration shall be replenished using one half the number of squeezes used initially (e.g., 5, 10 or 15).

(10) The test subject shall indicate to the test conductor if at any time during the fit test the taste of Bitrex is detected. If the test subject does not report tasting the Bitrex, the test is passed.

(11) If the taste of Bitrex is detected, the fit is deemed unsatisfactory and the test is failed. A different respirator shall be tried and the entire test procedure is repeated (taste threshold screening and fit testing).

5. Irritant Smoke (Stannic Chloride) Protocol

This qualitative fit test uses a person's response to the irritating chemicals released in the "smoke" produced by a stannic chloride ventilation smoke tube to detect leakage into the respirator.

(a) General Requirements and Precautions

(1) The respirator to be tested shall be equipped with high efficiency particulate air (HEPA) or P100 series filter(s).

(2) Only stannic chloride smoke tubes shall be used for this protocol.

(3) No form of test enclosure or hood for the test subject shall be used.

(4) The smoke can be irritating to the eyes, lungs, and nasal passages. The test conductor shall take precautions to minimize the test subject's exposure to irritant smoke. Sensitivity varies, and certain individuals may respond to a greater degree to irritant smoke. Care shall be taken when performing the sensitivity screening checks that determine whether the test subject can detect irritant smoke to use only the minimum amount of smoke necessary to elicit a response from the test subject.

(5) The fit test shall be performed in an area with adequate ventilation to prevent exposure of the person conducting the fit test or the build-up of irritant smoke in the general atmosphere.

(b) Sensitivity Screening Check

The person to be tested must demonstrate his or her ability to detect a weak concentration of the irritant smoke.

(1) The test operator shall break both ends of a ventilation smoke tube containing stannic chloride, and attach one end of the smoke tube to a low flow air pump set to deliver 200 milliliters per minute, or an aspirator squeeze bulb. The test operator shall cover the other end of the smoke tube with a short piece of tubing to prevent potential injury from the jagged end of the smoke tube.

(2) The test operator shall advise the test subject that the smoke can be irritating to the eyes, lungs, and nasal passages and instruct the subject to keep his/her eyes closed while the test is performed.

(3) The test subject shall be allowed to smell a weak concentration of the irritant smoke before the respirator is donned to become familiar with its irritating properties and to determine if he/she can detect the irritating properties of the smoke. The test operator

shall carefully direct a small amount of the irritant smoke in the test subject's direction to determine that he/she can detect it.

(c) Irritant Smoke Fit Test Procedure

(1) The person being fit tested shall don the respirator without assistance, and perform the required user seal check(s).
(2) The test subject shall be instructed to keep his/her eyes closed.

(3) The test operator shall direct the stream of irritant smoke from the smoke tube toward the faceseal area of the test subject, using the low flow pump or the squeeze bulb. The test operator shall begin at least 12 inches from the facepiece and move the smoke stream around the whole perimeter of the mask. The operator shall gradually make two more passes around the perimeter of the mask, moving to within six inches of the respirator.

(4) If the person being tested has not had an involuntary response and/or detected the irritant smoke, proceed with the test exercises.

(5) The exercises identified in section I A. 14. of this appendix shall be performed by the test subject while the respirator seal is being continually challenged by the smoke, directed around the perimeter of the respirator at a distance of six inches.

(6) If the person being fit tested reports detecting the irritant smoke at any time, the test is failed. The person being retested must repeat the entire sensitivity check and fit test procedure.

(7) Each test subject passing the irritant smoke test without evidence of a response (involuntary cough, irritation) shall be given a second sensitivity screening check, with the smoke from the same smoke tube used during the fit test, once the respirator has been removed, to determine whether he/she still reacts to the smoke. Failure to evoke a response shall void the fit test.

(8) If a response is produced during this second sensitivity check, then the fit test is passed.

C. Quantitative Fit Test (QNFT) Protocols

The following quantitative fit testing procedures have been demonstrated to be acceptable: Quantitative fit testing using a non-hazardous test aerosol (such as corn oil, polyethylene glycol 400 [PEG 400], di-2-ethyl hexyl sebacate [DEHS], or sodium chloride) generated in a test chamber, and employing instrumentation to quantify the fit of the respirator; Quantitative fit testing using ambient aerosol as the test agent and appropriate instrumentation (condensation nuclei counter) to quantify the respirator fit; Quantitative fit testing using controlled negative pressure and appropriate instrumentation to measure the volumetric leak rate of a facepiece to quantify the respirator fit.

1. General

(a) The employer shall ensure that persons administering QNFT are able to calibrate equipment and perform tests properly, recognize invalid tests, calculate fit factors properly and ensure that test equipment is in proper working order.

(b) The employer shall ensure that QNFT equipment is kept clean, and is maintained and calibrated according to the manufacturer's instructions so as to operate at the parameters for which it was designed.

2. Generated Aerosol Quantitative Fit Testing Protocol

(a) Apparatus.

(1) Instrumentation. Aerosol generation, dilution, and measurement systems using particulates (corn oil, polyethylene glycol 400 [PEG 400], di-2-ethyl hexyl sebacate [DEHS] or sodium chloride) as test aerosols shall be used for quantitative fit testing.

(2) Test chamber. The test chamber shall be large enough to permit all test subjects to perform freely all required exercises without disturbing the test agent concentration or the measurement apparatus. The test chamber shall be equipped and constructed so that the test agent is effectively isolated from the ambient air, yet uniform in concentration throughout the chamber.

(3) When testing air-purifying respirators, the normal filter or cartridge element shall be replaced with a high efficiency particulate air (HEPA) or P100 series filter supplied by the same manufacturer.

(4) The sampling instrument shall be selected so that a computer record or strip chart record may be made of the test showing the rise and fall of the test agent concentration with each inspiration and expiration at fit factors of at least 2,000. Integrators or computers that integrate the amount of test agent penetration leakage into the respirator for each exercise may be used provided a record of the readings is made.

(5) The combination of substitute air-purifying elements, test agent and test agent concentration shall be such that the test subject is not exposed in excess of an established exposure limit for the test agent at any time during the testing process, based upon the length of the exposure and the exposure limit duration.

(6) The sampling port on the test specimen respirator shall be placed and constructed so that no leakage occurs around the port (e.g., where the respirator is probed), a free air flow is allowed into the sampling line at all times, and there is no interference with the fit or performance of the respirator. The in-mask sampling device (probe) shall be designed and used so that the air sample is drawn from the breathing zone of the test subject, midway between the nose and mouth and with the probe extending into the facepiece cavity at least 1/4 inch.

(7) The test setup shall permit the person administering the test to observe the test subject inside the chamber during the test.

(8) The equipment generating the test atmosphere shall maintain the concentration of test agent constant to within a 10 percent variation for the duration of the test.

(9) The time lag (interval between an event and the recording of the event on the strip chart or computer or integrator) shall be kept to a minimum. There shall be a clear association between the occurrence of an event and its being recorded.

(10) The sampling line tubing for the test chamber atmosphere and for the respirator sampling port shall be of equal diameter and of the same material. The length of the two lines shall be equal.

(11) The exhaust flow from the test chamber shall pass through an appropriate filter (i.e , high efficiency particulate filter) before release.

(12) When sodium chloride aerosol is used, the relative humidity inside the test chamber shall not exceed 50 percent.

(13) The limitations of instrument detection shall be taken into account when determining the fit factor.

(14) Test respirators shall be maintained in proper working order and be inspected regularly for deficiencies such as cracks or missing valves and gaskets.

(b) Procedural Requirements.

(1) When performing the initial user seal check using a positive or negative pressure check, the sampling line shall be crimped closed in order to avoid air pressure leakage during either of these pressure checks.

(2) The use of an abbreviated screening QLFT test is optional. Such a test may be utilized in order to quickly identify poor fitting respirators that passed the positive and/or negative pressure test and reduce the amount of QNFT time. The use of the CNC QNFT instrument in the count mode is another optional method to obtain a quick estimate of fit and eliminate poor fitting respirators before going on to perform a full QNFT.

(3) A reasonably stable test agent concentration shall be measured in the test chamber prior to testing. For canopy or shower curtain types of test units, the determination of the test agent's stability may be established after the test subject has entered the test environment.

(4) Immediately after the subject enters the test chamber, the test agent concentration inside the respirator shall be measured to ensure that the peak penetration does not exceed 5 percent for a half mask or 1 percent for a full facepiece respirator.

(5) A stable test agent concentration shall be obtained prior to the actual start of testing.

(6) Respirator restraining straps shall not be over-tightened for testing. The straps shall be adjusted by the wearer without assistance from other persons to give a reasonably comfortable fit typical of normal use. The respirator shall not be adjusted once the fit test exercises begin.

(7) The test shall be terminated whenever any single peak penetration exceeds 5 percent for half masks and 1 percent for full facepiece respirators. The test subject shall be refitted and retested.

(8) Calculation of fit factors.

(i) The fit factor shall be determined for the quantitative fit test by taking the ratio of the average chamber concentration to the concentration measured inside the respirator for each test exercise except the grimace exercise.

(ii) The average test chamber concentration shall be calculated as the arithmetic average of the concentration measured before and after each test (i.e., 7 exercises) or the arithmetic average of the concentration measured before and after each exercise or the true average measured continuously during the respirator sample.

(iii) The concentration of the challenge agent inside the respirator shall be determined by one of the following methods:

(A) Average peak penetration method means the method of determining test agent penetration into the respirator utilizing a strip chart recorder, integrator, or computer. The agent penetration is determined by an average of the peak heights on the graph or by computer integration, for each exercise except the grimace exercise. Integrators or computers that calculate the actual test agent penetration into the respirator for each exercise will also be considered to meet the requirements of the average peak penetration method.

(B) Maximum peak penetration method means the method of determining test agent penetration in the respirator as determined by strip chart recordings of the test. The highest peak penetration for a given exercise is taken to be representative of average penetration into the respirator for that exercise.

(C) Integration by calculation of the area under the individual peak for each exercise except the grimace exercise. This includes computerized integration.

(D) The calculation of the overall fit factor using individual exercise fit factors involves first converting the exercise fit factors to penetration values, determining the average, and then converting that result back to a fit factor. This procedure is described in the following equation:

$$\text{Overall Fit Factor} = \frac{\text{Number of exercises}}{1/ff_1 + 1/ff_2 + 1/ff_3 + 1/ff_4 + 1/ff_5 + 1/ff_6 + 1/ff_7 + 1/ff_8}$$

here ff_1, ff_2, ff_3, etc. are the fit factors for exercises 1, 2, 3, etc.

(9) The test subject shall not be permitted to wear a half mask or quarter facepiece respirator unless a minimum fit factor of 100 is obtained, or a full facepiece respirator unless a minimum fit factor of 500 is obtained.

(10) Filters used for quantitative fit testing shall be replaced whenever increased breathing resistance is encountered, or when the test agent has altered the integrity of the filter media.

3. Ambient aerosol condensation nuclei counter (CNC) quantitative fit testing protocol.

The ambient aerosol condensation nuclei counter (CNC) quantitative fit testing (Portacount ™) protocol quantitatively fit tests respirators with the use of a probe. The probed respirator is only used for quantitative fit tests. A probed respirator has a special sampling device, installed on the respirator, that allows the probe to sample the air from inside the mask. A probed respirator is required for each make, style, model, and size that the employer uses and can be obtained from the respirator manufacturer or distributor. The CNC instrument manufacturer, TSI Inc., also provides probe attachments (TSI sampling adapters) that permit fit testing in an employee's own respirator. A minimum fit factor pass level of at least 100 is necessary for a half-mask respirator and a minimum fit factor pass level of at least 500 is required for a full facepiece negative pressure respirator. The entire screening and testing procedure shall be explained to the test subject prior to the conduct of the screening test.

(a) Portacount Fit Test Requirements.

(1) Check the respirator to make sure the sampling probe and line are properly attached to the facepiece and that the respirator is fitted with a particulate filter capable of preventing significant penetration by the ambient particles used for the fit test (e.g., NIOSH 42 CFR 84 series 100, series 99, or series 95 particulate filter) per manufacturer's instruction.

(2) Instruct the person to be tested to don the respirator for five minutes before the fit test starts. This purges the ambient particles trapped inside the respirator and permits the wearer to make certain the respirator is comfortable. This individual shall already have been trained on how to wear the respirator properly.

(3) Check the following conditions for the adequacy of the respirator fit: Chin properly placed; Adequate strap tension, not overly tightened; Fit across nose bridge; Respirator of proper size to span distance from nose to chin; Tendency of the respirator to slip; Self-observation in a mirror to evaluate fit and respirator position.

(4) Have the person wearing the respirator do a user seal check. If leakage is detected, determine the cause. If leakage is from a poorly fitting facepiece, try another size of the same model respirator, or another model of respirator.

(5) Follow the manufacturer's instructions for operating the Portacount and proceed with the test.

(6) The test subject shall be instructed to perform the exercises in section I. A. 14. of this appendix.

(7) After the test exercises, the test subject shall be questioned by the test conductor regarding the comfort of the respirator upon completion of the protocol. If it has become unacceptable, another model of respirator shall be tried.

(b) Portacount Test Instrument.

(1) The Portacount will automatically stop and calculate the overall fit factor for the entire set of exercises. The overall fit factor is what counts. The Pass or Fail message will indicate whether or not the test was successful. If the test was a Pass, the fit test is over.

(2) Since the pass or fail criterion of the Portacount is user programmable, the test operator shall ensure that the pass or fail criterion meet the requirements for minimum respirator performance in this Appendix.

(3) A record of the test needs to be kept on file, assuming the fit test was successful. The record must contain the test subject's name; overall fit factor; make, model, style, and size of respirator used; and date tested.

4. Controlled negative pressure (CNP) quantitative fit testing protocol.

The CNP protocol provides an alternative to aerosol fit test methods. The CNP fit test method technology is based on exhausting air from a temporarily sealed respirator facepiece to generate and then maintain a constant negative pressure inside the facepiece. The rate of air exhaust is controlled so that a constant negative pressure is maintained in the respirator during the fit test. The level of pressure is selected to replicate the mean inspiratory pressure that causes leakage into the respirator under normal use conditions. With pressure held constant, air flow out of the respirator is equal to air flow into the respirator. Therefore, measurement of the exhaust stream that is required to hold the pressure in the temporarily sealed respirator constant yields a direct measure of leakage air flow into the respirator. The CNP fit test method measures leak rates through the facepiece as a method for determining the facepiece fit for negative pressure respirators. The CNP instrument manufacturer Occupational Health Dynamics of Birmingham, Alabama also provides attachments (sampling manifolds) that replace the filter cartridges to permit fit testing in an employee's own respirator. To perform the test, the test subject closes his or her mouth and holds his/her breath, after which an air pump removes air from the respirator facepiece at a pre-selected constant pressure. The facepiece fit is expressed as the leak rate through the facepiece, expressed as milliliters per minute. The quality and validity of the CNP fit tests are determined by the degree to which the in-mask pressure tracks the test pressure during the system measurement time of approximately five seconds. Instantaneous feedback in the form of a real-time pressure trace of the in-mask pressure is provided and used to determine test validity and quality. A minimum fit factor pass level of 100 is necessary for a half-mask respirator and a minimum fit factor of at least 500 is required for a full facepiece respirator. The entire screening and testing procedure shall be explained to the test subject prior to the conduct of the screening test.

(a) CNP Fit Test Requirements.

(1) The instrument shall have a non-adjustable test pressure of 15.0 mm water pressure.

(2) The CNP system defaults selected for test pressure shall be set at ~ 15 mm of water (-0.58 inches of water) and the modeled inspiratory flow rate shall be 53.8 liters per minute for performing fit tests.

(Note: CNP systems have built-in capability to conduct fit testing that is specific to unique work rate, mask, and gender situations that might apply in a specific workplace. Use of system default values, which were selected to represent respirator wear with medium cartridge resistance at a low-moderate work rate, will allow inter-test comparison of the respirator fit.)

(3) The individual who conducts the CNP fit testing shall be thoroughly trained to perform the test.

(4) The respirator filter or cartridge needs to be replaced with the CNP test manifold. The inhalation valve downstream from the manifold either needs to be temporarily removed or propped open.

(5) The employer must train the test subject to hold his or her breath for at least 10 seconds.

(6) The test subject must don the test respirator without any assistance from the test administrator who is conducting the CNP fit test. The respirator must not be adjusted once the fit-test exercises begin. Any adjustment voids the test, and the test subject must repeat the fit test.

(7) The QNFT protocol shall be followed according to section I. C. 1. of this appendix with an exception for the CNP test exercises.

(b) CNP Test Exercises.

(1) Normal breathing. In a normal standing position, without talking, the subject shall breathe normally for 1 minute. After the normal breathing exercise, the subject needs to hold head straight ahead and hold his or her breath for 10 seconds during the test measurement.

(2) Deep breathing. In a normal standing position, the subject shall breathe slowly and

deeply for 1 minute, being careful not to hyperventilate. After the deep breathing exercise, the subject shall hold his or her head straight ahead and hold his or her breath for 10 seconds during test measurement.

(3) Turning head side to side. Standing in place, the subject shall slowly turn his or her head from side to side between the extreme positions on each side for 1 minute. The head shall be held at each extreme momentarily so the subject can inhale at each side. After the turning head side to side exercise, the subject needs to hold head full left and hold his or her breath for 10 seconds during test measurement. Next, the subject needs to hold head full right and hold his or her breath for 10 seconds during test measurement.

(4) Moving head up and down. Standing in place, the subject shall slowly move his or her head up and down for 1 minute. The subject shall be instructed to inhale in the up position (i.e., when looking toward the ceiling). After the moving head up and down exercise, the subject shall hold his or her head full up and hold his or her breath for 10 seconds during test measurement. Next, the subject shall hold his or her head full down and hold his or her breath for 10 seconds during test measurement.

(5) Talking. The subject shall talk out loud slowly and loud enough so as to be heard clearly by the test conductor. The subject can read from a prepared text such as the Rainbow Passage, count backward from 100, or recite a memorized poem or song for 1 minute. After the talking exercise, the subject shall hold his or her head straight ahead and hold his or her breath for 10 seconds during the test measurement.

(6) Grimace. The test subject shall grimace by smiling or frowning for 15 seconds.

(7) Bending Over. The test subject shall bend at the waist as if he or she were to touch his or her toes for 1 minute. Jogging in place shall be substituted for this exercise in those test environments such as shroud-type QNFT units that prohibit bending at the waist. After the bending over exercise, the subject shall hold his or her head straight ahead and hold his or her breath for 10 seconds during the test measurement.

(8) Normal Breathing. The test subject shall remove and re-don the respirator within a one-minute period. Then, in a normal standing position, without talking, the subject shall breathe normally for 1 minute. After the normal breathing exercise, the subject shall hold his or her head straight ahead and hold his or her breath for 10 seconds during the test measurement. After the test exercises, the test subject shall be questioned by the test conductor regarding the comfort of the respirator upon completion of the protocol. If it has become unacceptable, another model of a respirator shall be tried.

(c) CNP Test Instrument.

(1) The test instrument must have an effective audio-warning device, or a visual-warning device in the form of a screen tracing, that indicates when the test subject fails to hold his or her breath during the test. The test must be terminated and restarted from the

beginning when the test subject fails to hold his or her breath during the test. The test subject then may be refitted and retested.

(2) A record of the test shall be kept on file, assuming the fit test was successful. The record must contain the test subject's name; overall fit factor; make, model, style and size of respirator used; and date tested.

5. Controlled negative pressure (CNP) REDON quantitative fit testing protocol.

(a) When administering this protocol to test subjects, employers must comply with the requirements specified in paragraphs (a) and (c) of Part I.C.4 of this appendix ("Controlled negative pressure (CNP) quantitative fit testing protocol"), as well as use the test exercises described below in paragraph (b) of this protocol instead of the test exercises specified in paragraph (b) of Part I.C.4 of this appendix.

(b) Employers must ensure that each test subject being fit tested using this protocol follows the exercise and measurement procedures, including the order of administration, described below in Table A-1 of this appendix.

Table A-1. – CNP REDON Quantitative Fit Testing Protocol

Exercises[1]	Exercise procedure	Measurement procedure
Facing Forward	Stand and breathe normally, without talking, for 30 seconds.	Face forward, while holding breath for 10 seconds.
Bending Over	Bend at the waist, as if going to touch his or her toes, for 30 seconds.	Face parallel to the floor, while holding breath for 10 seconds
Head Shaking	For about three seconds, shake head back and forth vigorously several times while shouting.	Face forward, while holding breath for 10 seconds.
REDON 1	Remove the respirator mask, loosen all facepiece straps, and then redon the respirator mask.	Face forward, while holding breath for 10 seconds.
REDON 2	Remove the respirator mask, loosen all facepiece straps, and then redon the respirator mask again.	Face forward, while holding breath for 10 seconds.

[1] Exercises are listed in the order in which they are to be administered.

(c) After completing the test exercises, the test administrator must question each test subject regarding the comfort of the respirator. When a test subject states that the respirator is unacceptable, the employer must ensure that the test administrator repeats the protocol using another respirator model.

(d) Employers must determine the overall fit factor for each test subject by calculating the harmonic mean of the fit testing exercises as follows:

$$\text{Overall Fit Factor} = \frac{N}{\left[1/FF_1 + 1/FF_2 + \ldots \; 1/FF_N \right]}$$

Where:
N = The number of exercises;
FF1 = The fit factor for the first exercise;
FF2 = The fit factor for the second exercise; and
FFN = The fit factor for the nth exercise.

Part II. New Fit Test Protocols

A. Any person may submit to OSHA an application for approval of a new fit test protocol. If the application meets the following criteria, OSHA will initiate a rulemaking proceeding under section 6(b)(7) of the OSH Act to determine whether to list the new protocol as an approved protocol in this Appendix A.

B. The application must include a detailed description of the proposed new fit test protocol. This application must be supported by either:

1. A test report prepared by an independent government research laboratory (e.g., Lawrence Livermore National Laboratory, Los Alamos National Laboratory, the National Institute for Standards and Technology) stating that the laboratory has tested the protocol and had found it to be accurate and reliable; or

2. An article that has been published in a peer-reviewed industrial hygiene journal describing the protocol and explaining how test data support the protocol's accuracy and reliability.

C. If OSHA determines that additional information is required before the Agency commences a rulemaking proceeding under this section, OSHA will so notify the applicant and afford the applicant the opportunity to submit the supplemental information. Initiation of a rulemaking proceeding will be deferred until OSHA has received and evaluated the supplemental information.

[63 FR 20098, April 23, 1998; 69 FR 46993, August 4, 2004]

APPENDIX B: APPENDIX B-1 OF OSHA RESPIRATORY PROTECTION STANDARD

Appendix B. Appendix B-1 to § 1910.134: User Seal Check Procedures (Mandatory)

The individual who uses a tight-fitting respirator is to perform a user seal check to ensure that an adequate seal is achieved each time the respirator is put on. Either the positive and negative pressure checks listed in this appendix, or the respirator manufacturer's recommended user seal check method shall be used. User seal checks are not substitutes for qualitative or quantitative fit tests.

I. Facepiece Positive and/or Negative Pressure Checks

A. *Positive pressure check.* Close off the exhalation valve and exhale gently into the facepiece. The face fit is considered satisfactory if a slight positive pressure can be built up inside the facepiece without any evidence of outward leakage of air at the seal. For most respirators this method of leak testing requires the wearer to first remove the exhalation valve cover before closing off the exhalation valve and then carefully replacing it after the test.

B. *Negative pressure check.* Close off the inlet opening of the canister or cartridge(s) by covering with the palm of the hand(s) or by replacing the filter seal(s), inhale gently so that the facepiece collapses slightly, and hold the breath for ten seconds. The design of the inlet opening of some cartridges cannot be effectively covered with the palm of the hand. The test can be performed by covering the inlet opening of the cartridge with a thin latex or nitrile glove. If the facepiece remains in its slightly collapsed condition and no inward leakage of air is detected, the tightness of the respirator is considered satisfactory.

II. Manufacturer's Recommended User Seal Check Procedures

The respirator manufacturer's recommended procedures for performing a user seal check may be used instead of the positive and/or negative pressure check procedures provided that the employer demonstrates that the manufacturer's procedures are equally effective.

[63 FR 1152, Jan. 8, 1998]

Acknowledgements and Availability of Report

The Respiratory Disease Hazard Evaluation and Technical Assistance Program (RDHETAP) of NIOSH conducts field investigations of possible health hazards in the workplace. These investigations are conducted under the authority of Section 20(a)(6) of the Occupational Safety and Health (OSH) Act of 1970, 29 U.S.C. 669(a)(6), or Section 501(a)(11) of the Federal Mine Safety and Health Act of 1977, 30 U.S.C. 951(a)(11), which authorizes the Secretary of Health and Human Services, following a written request from any employers or authorized representative of employees, to determine whether any substance normally found in the place of employment has potentially toxic effects in such concentrations as used or found.

RDHETAP also provides, upon request, technical and consultative assistance to federal, state, and local agencies; labor; industry; and other groups or individuals to control occupational health hazards and to prevent related trauma and disease.

Mention of any company or product does not constitute endorsement by NIOSH. In addition, citations to websites external to NIOSH do not constitute NIOSH endorsement of the sponsoring organizations or their programs or products. Furthermore, NIOSH is not responsible for the content of these websites. All web addresses referenced in this document were accessible as of the publication date.

This report was prepared by Randy Boylstein, Rachel Bailey, Chris Piacitelli, Christine Schuler, Jean Cox-Ganser, and Kathleen Kreiss of the Field Studies Branch, Division of Respiratory Disease Studies. Desktop publishing was performed by Tia McClelland. We acknowledge David Brittain, Anne Marie Gibson, Kimberlee Musser, Brenda Naizby, Dianna Schoonmaker-Bopp, and Erin Spier, New York State Department of Health; and Johannes Peters, Sally Wheeland, Marilyn Reynolds, and Justin Lewis, county health department.

Copies of this report have been sent to the shredding facility, local county health department, New York State Department of Health, and the OSHA Regional Office. This report is not copyrighted and may be freely reproduced. The report may be viewed and printed at www.cdc.gov/niosh/hhe/. Copies may be purchased from the National Technical Information Service (NTIS) at 5825 Port Royal Road, Springfield, Virginia 22161.